5-13: A MEMOIR OF
LOVE, LOSS AND SURVIVAL

5-13: A MEMOIR OF LOVE, LOSS AND SURVIVAL

NANCY RANKIE SHELTON

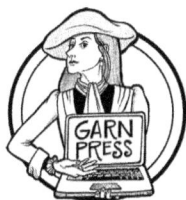

GARN PRESS

NEW YORK, NY

Published by Garn Press, LLC
New York, NY
www.garnpress.com

Book and cover design by Benjamin J. Taylor/Garn Press

Library of Congress Control Number: 2016933181

Publisher's Cataloging-in-Publication Data

Names: Shelton, Nancy Rankie.
Title: 5-13 : a memoir of love, loss and survival / Nancy Rankie Shelton.
Description: New York : Garn Press, 2016
Identifiers: LCCN 2016933181 | ISBN 978-1-942146-35-3 (pbk.) | ISBN 978-1-942146-36-0 (hardcover) | ISBN 978-1-942146-37-7 (ebook)
Subjects: LCSH: Lungs--Cancer--Patients--Biography. | Lungs--Cancer--Patients--Family States--Citizen participation. | Public schools--United States. |relationships. | Women caregivers--Biography | Caregivers' writings. | BISAC: BIOGRAPHY & AUTOBIOGRAPHY / Personal Memoirs. | FAMILY & RELATIONSHIPS / Death, Grief, Bereavement. | FAMILY & RELATIONSHIPS / Marriage & Long Term Relationships. | HEALTH & FITNESS / Diseases / Cancer.
Classification: LCC RC265.6 S53 2016 (print) | LCC RC265.6 (ebook) | DDC 362.196/9940092--dc23.

To my son Conrad

through whom Jack continues to live and to love

and

To my parents C. Jane and Charles Rankie

whose devotion to each other served as a model for Jack and me

for life's not a paragraph
And death i think is no parenthesis

e.e. cummings

Contents

Author's Note

Writing this book has allowed me to look back and to relive my experience with Jack's cancer. To commit to memory our lives, all that was good and all that was difficult. In so doing, I feel released to now put my energy into finding a way to keep living, not merely to go through the motions we generally call life, but to build new paths and to create a new happiness.

This book is completely nonfiction. The events were recorded as they were lived and are retold using the present tense so that the readers are able to feel and know only what I felt and knew at the time the events took place. The dialogue was either recorded during the interactions in which they are presented or recreated from memory. There are no composite characters. The names of all health care providers who are not also personal friends have been changed. All other characters, the medical facilities, and locations for various events that took place have not been changed. The chronology of events as it is presented in the text is as it was lived.

While writing this book I conducted interviews with a number of people who were part of the events described, however, the story is told through my eyes only. I have been as accurate as possible, with a conscious effort to be as generous as I could possibly be to all the people who are part of the story while still holding true to the experiences as I lived them. It is easy to look back now and better understand various decisions that were made, but to tell the story of the five months, thirteen days Jack was under their collective care in retrospect would not offer the reader the same experience as the one that we lived. The doubt, frustration and uncertainty that we felt were important parts of our lives and are shared as part of this memoir.

I hope this book offers others a chance to live their lives more fully and to realize that the struggles they may face are struggles they can manage. I hope it helps people to understand the multiple ways in which life changes when a loved one is diagnosed with cancer, and, in turn, that there are multiple ways in which we can offer them our support.

CHAPTER ONE

Terrible Tuesday

2011

Tuesday, December 27

I see all of him. His broad shoulders. His jeans sagging off his slim hips. His unshaven face. The Gator mug in his hand. His smile. Those killer blue eyes.

"Are you feeling as good as I am?" he asks.

We both love these slow mornings. The kids are back at work after a few days off to celebrate Christmas. The temperatures are moderate. We have the French doors open, exposing us to the vast green of our back yard. Few kids live in the neighborhood so, unlike our home in Baltimore, we hear birds chirping instead of children playing.

"Yea, I am. I love it when we have time alone together," I say, my computer resting on my lap.

"Me too. It feels great to be back home."

"You don't have to remind me Mr. Florida Boy. 'Born with sand between your toes.' I know."

"I've just finished reading the paper. I'm getting ready to wash the car."

I'm not surprised Jack has his morning planned out. Even during our vacations, he maintains a routine. "Ha. So my dad got to you did he?" We had driven to Sun City Center to celebrate Jack's 58th birthday, which falls so close to Christmas that it's usually just given a nod, and Christmas with my parents and to show them our new car. In their usual banter, my father had pointed out the dead bugs on the grill, inevitable when one drives Florida highways for any distance.

"Yea, but he's right. We don't want to let those bug guts ruin the paint." Jack smiles as he admits this. He and my father have a relationship based on teasing. They get their messages across to each other with a few jokes. A few challenges. Even a dare here and there.

We hadn't really planned to buy a new car during this trip, but with our sights set on retiring and returning to live in this house in a few years it seemed like a good time to trade in our aging SUV. I was able to convince Jack that I wanted a car again, no pick up truck, no SUV. Just a plain old car. We've not owned a *car* for about two decades.

But we didn't get a plain old car, instead we treated ourselves to a Mercedes Benz, something I've always dreamed of owning – never believing I would. We stumbled upon a great "deal" on a 2006 CLS 500 and negotiated the trade-in just two days before Christmas.

"How's your grading going?"

"It's going." I set my computer on the chair's arm and watch Jack. He's not a leaner or one to sit down very often. He's still standing, weight balanced evenly on both feet in a stance left over from his days in military boarding school. He's got that twinkle in his eyes that I know means he's going to tempt me away from my work.

Grinning, he says, "I see you didn't shower yet. Wait for me. We'll shower together after I finish the car."

I can't stop myself from matching his grin. I feel young again, sneaking sex when Conrad's not home. "You know I'll wait. That's the best invitation I've had all day."

Our friends typically spend their vacations surfing in Costa Rica, skiing in Colorado, or squandering their money in Las Vegas. When Jack and I are away from Maryland we almost always come to Gainesville to spend time with our son Conrad, his wife Kiley, and each other. When we left Florida in 2003 for me to start a position teaching in higher education, we decided to keep our home in Florida. After a few years, we sold the home where we had raised Conrad, and bought this house, in a golf course community, where we plan to live when we retire. Conrad and his wife Kiley live in the house now, which is a perfect arrangement for all of us.

Semester breaks are not a "vacation" for a full time professor. I keep up with the demands of my job, spending time each day grading, analyzing data and writing reports, or revising my syllabus for the upcoming semester. Jack is not faculty, he's a research scientist. He stays in touch with his colleagues in the lab, but when he's away, he really is on vacation. He uses the time to catch up on weeding, trimming the hedges, and making the constantly needed repairs to our sprinkler system. He has a 15-foot Stott Craft fishing boat, and he putters around keeping it in good running order. Once the boat's batteries are charged and Jack's made sure its motor is fine, we always spend a few days on Lake Sante Fe. No trip to Florida is complete without a drive to Crystal River where we swim with the manatees and spend time with our friends, Pat and Sue.

It's not just the sunshine, cloudless skies and inviting waterways everyone associates with Florida that draw us to return every chance we get. We long for the spacious landscapes, green environment (not politically green but grass, trees, gardens), single-family homes, and roads lined with sidewalks. Gainesville is quite a contrast to Baltimore, where our other home is, where multi-story buildings block out any sunlight that might escape through the ever-clouded sky.

Jack ambles out of the study and disappears around the corner heading to the other end of the house. It's quiet again. I easily sink back into my work. I'm making good progress and quickly put myself back in the "zone" and focus on the task at hand, shutting out the world around me. The semester's end always means mountains of mental work. It's not just about "grading papers" but the much more important work of reflection. Questions such as *What did my students learn? How well did they understand the theoretical foundations of literacy development?* and *What adjustments will I need to make next semester?* are constantly in the forefront of my mind.

I work for another hour before I'm slowly dragged out of my zone, realizing the dogs are barking too loud and too long. I turn my head towards the study door to hear better, wondering, *Where is Jack? Why is he not responding to Gus and Juno?* I continue to listen and realize there's another sound coming from somewhere. It's a guttural cry. My hearing impairment disallows me to identify the sound. It's getting louder. I start to panic. I thrust my computer off my lap onto the floor and run out of the study calling out to Jack. "Where are you? Jack, what's wrong? Why are you making that sound?"

The only responses are the dogs' continued barking and an odd human-like sound I can't identify. My hearing is unilateral and I can't tell the direction of the sound. I run from room to room looking for Jack. After circling the house twice my fear turns to panic. I force myself to stop running. Standing motionless in the hallway, I ask myself, *How will I find Jack?* As soon as I stop, I realize the dogs are right by me barking and will lead me to the noise, to Jack, if I let them. I follow them back into the kitchen where I had already been but hadn't seen Jack. Within seconds, Gus is standing next to Jack, who is lying on the floor.

I run to Jack. He's flat on the floor, his body stiff but one hand is above his chest, shaking. Not knowing at all what to do, I sink down beside him and start pounding his chest because I think he might be having a heart attack and I don't want his heart to stop. Crying out, "Don't you dare die on me Jack. Oh my God Jack, you can't leave me. Don't you dare die." I watch him long enough to know this isn't a heart attack, but some kind of seizure.

I run back to the study to grab my cell phone. I dial 911 as I run back to the kitchen. I put the phone to my ear. There's no sound. I can't hear anything. *Damn! The Bluetooth is on and it's still in the study where I was working.* I rush back to the study, grab my Bluetooth as fast as I can and hurry back to Jack. He's still seizing.

Finally. "911. What is your emergency?"

"My husband is having a seizure or a heart attack or something. I need help."

"Are you with him?"

"Yes."

"Is he conscious?"

Jack's hand finally stops shaking and he's able to speak. I tell the dispatcher everything Jack tells me. Jack was washing the car when he felt stroke-like symptoms. He explains to me, and I to the dispatcher, that he was able to negotiate himself back into the house, but only with great difficulty. He first felt his hand curl into his body, then his facial muscles pulled down making speech impossible, then his right leg became stiff and finally his left leg did the same. With deliberate determination he was able to get to the kitchen counter, which he leaned over to lower himself down onto the floor so he wouldn't fall. Though he couldn't speak because he was seizing, he cried out to me for help – that was the guttural sound that finally jolted me away from my work.

The dispatcher asks a series of questions. Jack can talk. He can think. He can tell the dispatcher his medical history better than I can.

After I get Gus and Juno in Conrad's bedroom and close the door, I open the front door so the medics will have immediate access to the house. I rush back to Jack.

The paramedics arrive. Jack is fully conscious and he has most of his body movement back under his own conscious control, but his right hand is paralyzed. He is stable enough for me to walk away while the EMTs examine him. I call Conrad. He's going to meet us at Shands Hospital at the University of Florida.

While the paramedics move Jack onto the stretcher I call my brother John to let him know something has happened to Jack – that he has had a seizure or stroke or something and we're on our way to the hospital. The paramedics are pushing Jack out of the front door just as our neighbor, Eric, walks up.

"Nancy, what can I do?" Eric asks.

I hand him my house key. "Please let the dogs out of the back room and lock the house after we leave."

"Of course. Here's my phone number. Call if you need anything."

I watch as the medics load Jack into the ambulance and then I climb in the cab next to the driver. Jack is stable again so there are no sirens, no lights – just a dreadfully silent ride to Shands.

As soon as the ambulance turns into the ER entrance, I see Kiley and Conrad. By the time I can climb out of the ambulance, the medics are already unloading Jack. Kiley and Conrad are next to me as Jack flashes Conrad a "thumbs up" to assure him he's okay.

Within a short time frame, neurologist, neurosurgeons and internal medicine physicians surround Jack. As the physicians try to sort out whether or not Jack has had a seizure or a stroke, they take him out of the ER bay to complete tests.

Kiley and Conrad are talking to another physician on the other side of the glass doors that close off Jack's ER bay. Conrad has his arm around Kiley's shoulders. They look intimately connected. I'm grateful they are here. I walk out of the little room, which feels cold and empty. Conrad hugs me. Feeling his warmth gives me strength.

Soon I see someone pushing Jack's bed back towards us. There are too many people in white coats moving in tandem with the bed. Jack, who just a few hours ago, was standing in our study in full control of his body, his direction, his decisions, now seems to be a miniature of himself, swallowed by white sheets, white coats, and white hospital walls.

The transport staff skillfully wheel Jack's bed into the ER bay, lock down the bed's wheels and turn to leave.

"Thanks guys," Jack calls out to them. The ever-cordial man showing his gratitude.

We slowly file into the ER bay. Only one person has anything in his hands. That must be the doctor. Yes, he's holding a clipboard. He's taking command of the room without voicing a single word.

He's a big man. He has dark hair and kind eyes. He rolls his stool up close to Jack, directly across from where I'm leaning on Jack's bed, trying to remain upright. My body is shaking. My stomach hurts. There is no stool for me. There is one empty chair but it's several feet from Jack's bed and I'm not leaving Jack's side. I feel tension in the quietness of everyone's movements. No one is speaking.

Kiley and Conrad position themselves behind me. I feel the warmth of their presence even though I can't see them. I grip the rails of the hospital bed. I squeeze hard to keep myself steady.

Jack reaches out and cups his left hand over my right. At first his skin, dried and cracked from the winter weather we left behind in Maryland, feels scratchy, but when he squeezes my hand all I feel is his love.

The doctor glances down at the report on his clipboard, focuses his gaze at Jack, and in a soft voice asks, "Is it okay to talk about the test results with everyone in the room?"

"Yes," Jack's voice is clear. "This is my family. They need to know whatever it is you have to say."

No amount of bedside manner is enough for the words spoken next.

Jack has lung cancer.

CHAPTER TWO

Coming Together

John Conrad Shelton, Sr., nicknamed "Shelly" during his time as a Sherman tank commander during WWII, was born in North Carolina but eventually settled on the Shelton farm in Greensville, Tennessee. He met and married his second wife, Geraldine "Jerry" Keiser, a nurse also serving in the war. They settled in St. Petersburg Beach, Florida. Shelly was a builder and St. Pete Beach was fertile ground for development.

Shelly had a child with his first wife, but when he and Jerry tried to start a family, Jerry couldn't conceive. They decided to adopt a child.

Jack was born on December 20, 1953, and immediately given up for adoption. The sum total of what he knows about his birth parents is that they were sixteen and seventeen years old, they were unwed, and one was a preacher's child. Every time I ask him if we can search for them, if only for a medical history, Jack always responds the same. "They gave me up once, why would I give them the chance to do it again?"

The courts required adopted babies to stay in foster care for six months before being placed with their adoptive families. Three months after the placement, the adoption could be finalized.

Jack moved into the Shelton home after the infant waiting period was satisfied. When Jack's parents went to court to finalize Jack's adoption, Jerry was pregnant. Jack's brother, Jeff, was born July 4, 1955.

Sandy blond hair that fell in soft curls during his youth, five feet, eleven inches tall as an adult, Irish white skin covered in freckles, blue eyes, thin Irish lips, Jack looks nothing like his brother Jeff, who carries the Shelton genes. They both have thick strong shoulders but any physical resemblance ends there. Jeff is a tad bit shorter than Jack, naturally blond, with skin that tans almost to olive. Jack burns to bright red after a short half hour in the sun.

Jack and his mother, now deceased, never shared a mother/son bond beyond the most formal. Jerry was an alcoholic and a chain smoker. Throughout Jack's childhood Jerry had, instead of her children, a cigarette in one hand and Seagram's VO and Tab in her other.

Jack never remembers hugging his mother as a young boy. He doesn't remember mother/son outings. He can't remember a single time when he sat on her lap. Instead he remembers Louise, their maid. Louise taught him how to cook, cared for him when he was in need, and talked to him about his friends, school, and sports. He remembers being shipped off to nursery school when he was just three years old, and in later years his mother scornfully calling him "Al Capone." He has no happy memories connected to his mother.

Shelly's relationship with Jack was quite different. They shared a love for the outdoors and spent a great deal of time together. Shelly took Jack to his hunting cabin for weekend trips. Jack developed a deep reverence for firearms, but as neither a child nor an adult has he enjoyed killing animals. Shelly had a beautiful forty foot Chris Craft – one of those elegant wooden boats. He taught Jack how to captain the boat, and they would fish and dive together often. Shelly got a small fishing boat for Jack and Jeff, which they could take out on their own. Any happiness Jack had as a Shelton offspring ended when his father died of scleroderma in 1964.

Jack's childhood was fraught with pain that stemmed from being raised by a neglectful mother, her alcoholism distorting every relationship in the Shelton home, and the untimely death of his beloved father. But there were good times. Jack chose to take the good from his past and shape his life as an adult in ways that reject his mother's negativity and emulate his father's joys. Jack's childhood home was on the waterfront. The Gulf of Mexico was his playground. An avid swimmer, water skier, and fisherman, to this day Jack is more at home on the water than he is on land. He's a southern gentleman descended from the tobacco farms of Tennessee and the sands of St. Petersburg Beach.

Appropriately, Jack and I met when a group of people got together to go night fishing. It was April 1977. The previous June, after graduating from SUNY Albany, I had moved from Upstate New York to Florida. I was chasing a romance that had begun the summer between my junior and senior year in college while I was living with my sister Carol and her husband in St. Petersburg Beach. All was well between my boyfriend and me for several months after I moved, but when we went our separate ways, my main reason for living in Florida ceased to exist. My sister had moved back to New York and I couldn't find a job that would lead to a career. I'd waitressed long enough. I decided to move back to my roots.

In order to save enough money to make the trip back home, I gave up my little beach cottage in Pass-A-Grille and moved in with a friend. Debbie lived in Belle Vista, the neighborhood in St. Pete Beach where Jack grew up. One afternoon while Debbie and I were playing in her yard with her two daughters, Dawn and Dana, a guy visiting Debbie's neighbor walked across the street, started a conversation, and invited me to go fishing with him on his friend's boat.

The guy's name was Jeff Shelton. I told him I wasn't interested in dating. Jeff said the other guys would all have girls with them, and he just didn't want to go solo. He assured me we could just go as friends.

I was planning to leave Florida and decided this was a good opportunity to go night fishing one more time, something I sure wouldn't be able to do in Upstate New York.

There were four guys on the boat and no other women. I was a bit angry. Jeff had said there would be other women as part of the group.

Jack was one of the four guys. Since moving to Florida, Jack was one of the few men I had met who was in college. He was gentle, polite, a microbiology major, and I spent the night talking to him.

I decided I might be interested in dating after all.

Soon Jack and I were seeing each other every weekend and my plans to move back to New York were put on hold. I needed more time in Florida. The time I was spending with Jack was fun, and I liked him more each time we got together. I got a job at a school in Tampa and moved to an apartment in Hyde Park. Jack was a student at the University of Florida in Gainesville. We took turns making the drive between Tampa and Gainesville. Our weekends were spent with our friends on the water, fishing, diving, waterskiing or just cruising out on the Gulf to swim.

Before moving to Florida I had only gone fishing once or twice with my father and brother. My former boyfriend and I had done a lot of fishing off the sea wall, especially at night after the bars closed. I had my own fishing pole, tackle and bait bucket but I can't say I was much of a fisherwoman. Forget diving, I couldn't even manage a mask and snorkel without choking in water.

Jack introduced me to an entirely new and different life. Saturday mornings Pat, Sue, Jack and I packed beer, snacks, sandwiches and bait and spent the day out on the Gulf, singing "I like mine with lettuce and tomatoes" along with Jimmy Buffet, downing the beers in the hot sun, navigating from place to place seeking the big catch.

I was never the one to reel in the catch, big or small. Jack would pass hints my way but they never worked. I found great satisfaction when I finally realized it was Sue who was the one who reeled in the best fish. Neither Pat nor Jack could keep up with her.

When we were off for a day of diving, I always packed my fishing gear because I was the poor sucker who had to stay with the boat. I never minded because Pat always had a stash of frozen squid for bait, though when everyone was fishing we used live bait, not a box of ugly, smelly squid. I used those days to hone my skills as a fisherwoman. I was more relaxed fishing alone with no onlookers to make me feel awkward.

As soon as the divers splashed off the side of Pat's twenty-five foot Mako, I'd strip down to my bikini, dig the squid out of the bait cooler, somehow manage to cut strips off the squid's arms and force my hook through the chunk of squid, and cast away. I really didn't want to catch anything because I didn't know one fish from another and certainly had no idea how I'd get one off my hook should I ever get one on, but I figured I had nothing to worry about because the whole process was so foreign to me I was sure I needed years to catch up to these Floridians.

I rarely even got a fish to bite but on one occasion I thought I had finally learned the trick. Jack had taught me that when I felt any pressure on my line I needed to lead the fish on, letting it nibble at my bait but not so that it gobbled my bait up and swam away. I needed to reel the line in just a little to get the fish to follow it, take a big gulp, and that would set the hook and I'd have a catch.

I felt the pressure. I raised the end of my pole like Jack had taught me, then lowered it to reel in the line so there was no slack. I felt the pressure again, so I raised my pole again. There was too much pressure; I knew I had hooked it. I struggled with the reel. *God, it must be a big one,* I thought. Then I felt it. *Snap.* My line was free. Loose, with no pressure whatsoever. *Damn. I'll never get this right.* The rest of the day not a single fish teased my line.

The divers surfaced. Jack showed off the yellowtail he had shot with his spear gun. Pat bragged about the grouper he brought up. Then, with their tanks stowed safely, cold beers in their hands, their catches iced down in the cooler, the guys sat back for a little pleasure time.

Jack started it. "How'd your fishing go?" he asked.

"Oh, it was okay." I didn't want to admit I had lost yet another fish. The only Yankee on the boat, I had taken enough abuse from these damn Crackers.

"Did you catch anything?"

"No, but I still enjoyed it."

"Did you even get any bites?" Jack pushed.

"Yea," I answered, curious about his continued questioning. Jack didn't usually nag me when I gave short answers. I turned towards Jack, shooting him a side-glance hoping to make eye contact so he'd realize I didn't want to talk about my failure in front of everyone.

As soon as our eyes met, Jack's face exploded in a smile and Pat broke out laughing.

"He's yanking your chain, Nancy." Pat chuckled. "Well, not really your chain – your line."

"What do you mean?" I asked.

"Jack was that big fish you thought you caught," Pat explained.

Seeing Jack's devilish grin was all I needed to know he had messed with my line, making me think I had hooked a fish, and then lost it.

No doubt, we partied in our younger years. Jack smoked his share of pot, though I never liked the high I got from smoking pot. I've always had an aversion for cigarettes. The smoke gives me a headache and besides that, to me the idea of sucking in smoke that will inevitably kill you is ignorant.

I never dated smokers. If I noticed an attractive guy and he had a cigarette in his hand, I'd immediately look away. I was rude to men who smoked. I didn't want them near me. I didn't kiss tobacco-flavored mouths.

Even from our earliest days together, Jack never smoked cigarettes in front of me. But eventually I found out that he did smoke them. And it's been a source of tension throughout our marriage, especially in our earlier years. When I would smell smoke on Jack's breath, I would scorn my mantra at him – "Yea. Keep smoking those cancer sticks. And when you're lying in the hospital dying of cancer don't expect me to sit by your side."

It's an addiction Jack hates. He quits, then starts again, then quits again.

In 2007 Jack was diagnosed with peripheral artery disease. His motivation to quit was stronger than ever after that. As far as I know, he was finally successful because it's been at least eight years since I've happened upon Jack with a cigarette or smelled smoke on his breath or clothes.

Could I really have known all these years that one day I would be where I am right now? Sitting in Shands ER. Surrounded by doctors explaining that a mass in Jack's lung has metastasized and already spread to his brain where he has several marble-sized lesions.

I'm numb.

We're assured the tumor is near the base of Jack's lung and easily reachable for extraction. I can't process what this means.

"The decisions of how to treat you won't be made by the ER team. You will be admitted and oncologists will handle your diagnosis and treatment," the big man on the small stool with wheels says to us.

All those times I begged Jack to stop smoking mean nothing now. What means everything is our love for each other and our determination to fight this disease together.

CHAPTER 3

Cancer

Wednesday, December 28

My experience dealing with a major health problem is just about nil and my knowledge base about lung cancer is not much greater. I know I have a lot of learning ahead of me. I feel like I've been transported to a barren, strange world where I don't speak the language or know the people or customs.

I search my mind for anything that might help. Somewhere in the network of thoughts swirling in my head I can hear my sister Carol telling me to "write everything down." I know she hasn't told me this since Jack's seizure because I can't talk on the phone. I don't want to speak to anyone. I have to conserve my listening skills, I have to save my brain cells. I have to stay alert, tuned in to Jack and what's happening around me. But still, I hear Carol and I am writing everything down.

Before the day would normally even start for me I'm beginning my training. It's 7:10 AM. The neurosurgeon is in our room explaining the course of treatment for the lesions in Jack's brain. It's something called radiosurgery. He says radiosurgery can be done as an outpatient and that once the radiosurgery is done, it can take up to two weeks to reduce the swelling in Jack's brain.

I don't know what radiosurgery is. Jack is calling it "cyber knife" so I know he knows more than I do about this, but that's not helping because Jack is interrupting the doctor who is trying to explain it. I find myself asking more questions than the doctor wants to answer, including what the treatment will be for Jack's lung lesion (I've already learned that a tumor is a lesion – the doctors seem to use these terms interchangeably). There will be a different team of doctors who will decide what to do about the tumor in Jack's lung, which won't happen until after they do a biopsy.

At 8:10 another doctor comes in. This one is a resident, Dr. Lewis, from the primary team. I don't know what that means. What's primary and what's secondary? Someone must have ordered the biopsy because Dr. Lewis says it's scheduled for tomorrow. But the other information Dr. Lewis shares seems conflicting to me, because an hour ago we were told that we don't know at all what the treatment for Jack's lung will be but now we're being told all about chemotherapy. Apparently, chemotherapies are varied – treatments can be anywhere from one to several weeks. I'm confused and glad I'm writing everything down.

Dr. Lewis leaves. Jack and I just look at each other and say nothing. I'm sure Jack is as confused as I am but that's only because he's the one who is sick. Jack has experience with the science of cancer and knows about these treatments because of his work as a genetic researcher. But he doesn't want to hear these doctors talk about long-term illness, he wants to know when his hand, which is still paralyzed, will start working again and when he can get back to work. When I watch him, one minute I see a healthy Jack and the next I see a very sick man.

I thank God we're at least in a private room. Last night when Jack was moved from the ER to the floor, he was first put in a two-bed room. I made the mistake of asking the nurse to bring a chair that could serve as a bed. I was told that since Jack didn't have a private room, I legally could not stay overnight with him.

I didn't budge. I didn't blink. I wasn't leaving. I would just sleep in the upright chair if I had to. But as soon as the activity on the floor died down and the doctors and nurses were not coming in to see Jack with every tick of the clock, I closed Jack's privacy curtains and climbed up into his bed with him. Unfortunately, or fortunately as it turned out, about 10 PM the man in the bed beside Jack called the nurse who stuck her head in to say goodnight to Jack and saw me in his bed with him. She looked as stunned as any nurse I've ever seen.

Jack smiled at me, "We're busted." Being busted turned out okay. The staff, knowing it's against regulations to have me even in the room all night (forget about in the bed) managed to find a private room and dragged us to it at about midnight.

At 10:45 AM the neurology team (4 of them) comes in to talk about managing Jack's seizures. The doctors use language that detaches the disease from the man, explaining once again (as if we didn't hear this yesterday in the ER) that Jack's is a "serious" cancer.

The brain lesions caused Jack's brain to swell and this led to the seizures. Yesterday the doctors said that the MRI showed either two or three lesions. Today, it's being confirmed as three.

The lesions are located between the white and gray matter and the left frontal parietal. *What does that mean?* I don't know and I don't have time to find out before the next doctor arrives. This time it's Dr. Jamail, from Internal Medicine. He's here to talk about the biopsy.

Dr. Jamail explains that the doctors from the radiology department (we have not met them yet) will "go in through" Jack's chest to collect cells that will be identified to determine what kind of cancer Jack has.

Jack is frustrated. He does this work at his lab. He's trying to let these doctors know that he understands DNA testing of tumors. Jack keeps butting in, repeating his knowledge of gene mutations, especially, EGFR and KRAS, trying to force the doctors to engage in a professional conversation with him.

I can't even intervene on Jack's behalf and push Dr. Jamail to answer Jack because I know nothing about gene mutations and cancer. Jack's research is in human genetics and the studies he's involved in are confidential. He talks about his work with me but not in great detail.

"I do this research in my lab. I work with one of the premier researchers in personalized medicine." Jack knows that genetic sequencing the DNA from the tumor identifies the mutations, and that finding known mutations will give them direction on how to treat the specific cancer.

"Most of us are moving towards personalized medicine, Mr. Shelton. We will be testing to see if your tumor has the mutations." Though Dr. Jamail is finally responding to Jack, he's still not showing Jack the respect he seeks.

"Do you know the work Alan Shuldiner at the University of Maryland, Baltimore is doing? I work in his lab. I sequence DNA and have for 30 years."

Because of his scientific understanding of human disease, Jack knows it's not possible to immediately know what his exact treatment will be. Dr. Jamail explains the general treatments for lung cancer:

1.   Surgery, but only if the tumor is small and the cancer has not spread – not for Jack because his cancer has already spread to his brain.

2.   A combination of chemo and radiation therapies.

3.   Nothing – if the cancer is very bad and "the patient" only has two to three months to live.

The patient? No wonder this man nor any of his underlings would listen to Jack's knowledge of personalized medicine. Clearly the doctors have already depersonalized Jack as "the patient" and not the man he is. Is this another one of their distancing language techniques? Well I hate to tell him but it's not working – the only *patient he could be talking about right now is Jack, so why doesn't he just say so? As if depersonalizing his language can possibly depersonalize Jack's disease.*

Dr. Jamail, who seems to be the head of this team speaks, repeating the phrase "no treatment is an option" at least three times. He stresses the severity of Jack's disease. His bias is evident to me. In his opinion, Jack is not a candidate for treatment at all. Because Jack's cancer has already spread, there's a lot of pressure for us to understand that they can't cure Jack's cancer, they can only manage it. How they ultimately decide to manage it will be up to the oncologists who we won't see until after the biopsy is completed.

Jack has lost the use of his right hand and has a stroke-like droop in his face. His speech is slurred. He's frustrated because he can't express himself very well and all these doctors just seem to add more and more stress for Jack to handle.

Although I don't understand some of what the doctors are telling us, I'm trying to let my intellectual brain overtake the emotional brain. Jack can't do that – he's stopping the doctors in mid-sentence to ask when he will get the use of his hand back and if he will be able to drive in three weeks, which is when we are scheduled to return to Maryland. When they explain to Jack that he may be treated with chemotherapy, Jack stops the doctor in mid-sentence to ask if he has about two to three days to still taste food. Sadness and an overwhelming desire to protect Jack crush me as I watch his mind wander all over the place. The doctors just keep explaining that he has much bigger problems to worry about than driving or eating.

More than one doctor has already told him he has only three to six months to live, and one even told him he "needs to get his affairs in order." They haven't allowed Jack to eat because of the biopsy. Because of the lack of communication between all these medical teams, the nurses gave Jack his Plavix, a medication to prevent blood clots, this morning. They can't do the biopsy but they won't change the "no eating" order either.

Oh my goodness, it doesn't stop. At 1:50 PM Dr. Webb from Radiology comes in to further explain the biopsy procedure. They'll take sample tissue from the mass that's in Jack's left lower lung lobe. The sample is the keystone for determining how to proceed and will be used to determine treatment. The mass is three to four centimeters

– not too big according to this doctor. Jack will be on his belly for the procedure, his vitals will be monitored, and he will receive two meds (for pain and relaxing). The doctors will use a small needle to get a core tissue sample. The most common complications include a small risk of bleeding and the possibility of getting air in the lung. Jack may cough up blood after the procedure, which takes 45-90 minutes. The anesthesia will wear off in four to six hours.

My stomach is tense all the time. I feel confused. Empty. Lost. I have a horrible headache coming on. I just want to find a way to make this nightmare stop, to alter the universe and to bring it under my personal control. In my altered universe I would freeze-frame the last twenty-four hours, erase them completely and rewrite the script.

Dr. Vogel, a third year resident, is here. She will be Jack's primary doctor who will coordinate all the subspecialists. She's young, smiling, attractive, and wearing a Notre Dame tee shirt. Her shirt reminds Jack and me that it's still college football bowl season. For a change we're talking about something I understand with one of these doctors – football. Besides that, Dr. Vogel knows Brady, a young man who grew up in Gainesville and then went to undergrad at Notre Dame. Brady and Conrad knew each other as young children and Jack and I know Brady's parents. I'm actually starting to relax and I'm able to completely understand everything Dr. Vogel tells us.

Generally, when cancer presents as a single lesion, it's operable. When there are multiple lesions (as in Jack's case) it's much more likely the doctors won't operate. Jack has a single lesion in his lung and multiple lesions in his brain.

I'm starting to realize that my confusion and lack of understanding about what we are told about Jack's cancer is not my fault. The various doctors have given us conflicting information. The ER doctors yesterday said Jack's tumor was in a very operable spot, leading us to believe surgery might be an option. However, when more tests were completed and the extent to which Jack's cancer has spread became known, those first decisions were simply set aside and new decisions were made.

Dr. Vogel also explains that the radiation will shrink the lesions and hopefully minimize their growth. As for the biopsy, the cell identification is quick but they will also send tissue for additional stains, which can take a lot longer. A pathology report usually takes two to three days minimum.

At 6:35 PM tonight, almost twelve hours after our first doctor visit, the last doctor makes her rounds. This time it's Dr. Yuan, a member of Dr. Pham's team. We haven't met Dr. Pham yet, but our interactions with Dr. Yuan are much more conversational than what we've had with other doctors. She's very thorough. Jack is going to be transferred to the Cancer Hospital and there he'll get a new team. Dr. Yuan won't be on that team. But tonight she can explain all she knows for us. And she does. A lot of what she tells us supports and elaborates what other doctors have already shared but much of the information is new.

1. Jack's kidney function is slightly above normal. It's possible this is due to dyes from all the tests but they will monitor Jack's kidneys.

2. There are 3 lesions in Jack's brain that are 1.1 to 1.2 cm.

3. Jack's team ordered a CT Scan of Jack's pelvis and abdomen, which should let us know if there's something causing Jack's slight discomfort in his hip he feels some mornings.

4. The team ordered Jack's transfer to the Cancer Center.

5. Jack's brain tumors will be treated first, the lung tumor treatment will follow with chemo.

6. Jack's cancer is Stage 4, or Event stage (I haven't heard this terminology before).

7. Jack has "Great" performance, which is how strong his baseline health is. Apparently this is an important factor that will play into treatment decisions.

8.   Longevity with metastatic brain disease is less than
     one year, especially if the cells are the more aggressive
     (or small cell). Small cell expectations are less than six
     months, six to twelve months if large. Longevity also
     depends on the cancer's aggressiveness after treatment –
     an extremely important indicator.

I feel like a Ping-Pong ball being batted around by all these
doctors. We had seven different teams/individuals in our room
today, each with their own store of information. People come and
go constantly. I wish I could see all of these groups of specialists as
working together toward a collective treatment plan centered on
Jack's cancer, but I can't. Instead I see them as individual interests
competing with each other for a lead role.

At this point we will just wait for the biopsy, which won't be
done until tomorrow at the soonest. It feels like years of waiting.
But the oncologists need the results before they can plan treatment.
So we know nothing about our options for treatment for Jack's lung
lesion. The neurosurgeons have determined that they will conduct
the radiosurgery (which I now know is a single blast of radiation to
shrink the lesions in Jack's brain) but of course, when that happens
depends on the successful biopsy procedure.

The only good thing about all these people and the constant
activity is that there is very little time alone in which Jack and I
would be talking to each other about *longevity*. There's a monologue
screaming in my brain with a repeated phrase but it's not something I want to say out loud to any of the people caring for Jack. *Six
months? Are you kidding? Six months? Six months! You must have
that wrong! Six months?*

Tonight I decide to send an email to my family to ask them not
to call me on the phone. I can't talk without crying. I fear breaking down. In my mind the most important thing is for me to stay
strong, to listen to all the doctors and record everything I can as they
share information with us, and to do my best to help Jack, Kiley and
Conrad through each day, each decision, each challenge. I feel like

I've been swallowed by a dark, cold world where I must find strength for the four of us. It may seem cruel to others, but nothing else is important. It's easier for me to control my emotions when I write as opposed to talking so I'll send emails to my family when I can.

Thursday, December 29

This morning Jack and I start the day with another walk. Yesterday we ventured outside our room but today we decide to explore even further, walking the same halls that lap around the nurses' station feels too limiting. Jack is super conscious of keeping himself mobile and I need the exercise too.

As we peek around corners at the end of our wing, we find two hallways that offer new "landscape" for us. The doors to the right lead to a new wing, which seems cheerful and updated. But Jack, always thinking about other people before himself, doesn't want to go that way. He's concerned we'll invade other patients' privacy, so we turn the opposite direction to see what's on the other side of the double doors to the left.

We discover a long hallway lined with windows. The bright light is welcoming and I feel as close to being outside as I've been since the short walk two days ago from the ambulance to the ER.

Suddenly Jack stops. I glance at him to see what's wrong. His face is grimacing. Panic rises up in me but Jack quickly calms me down, "It's okay, it's just my hip. I felt this a few times in Baltimore when I was walking from the parking garage to my lab. I can walk it out." But when we try to step forward, Jack grabs the railing on the wall and stops again. He assures me he's okay and tries squatting down. I'm amazed at Jack. Here he's newly diagnosed with cancer, a seizure that put him on the floor and numbed his hand, and he can still squat better than I've been able to do since the late 1990s. Jack has made an effort to stay physically fit. He maintains his weight at 180 pounds, still has thin hips and strong shoulders that hint at his younger days as an avid sportsman.

All the squatting and stretching doesn't help. Jack's primary care doctor in Baltimore, Dr. Weaver, said these incidents of hip pain are probably the onset of arthritis, but whatever it is, I have to hold onto Jack and help him back to our room. I know he's in a lot of pain because he's really leaning on me. I'm relieved when we finally stumble back to safety.

At 8:50 Dr. Vogel, who we met yesterday, steps in. She reiterates what we were previously told – that Dr. Pham is the attending medical oncologist. She also reassures us that Jack can continue his care here at Shands for as long as we want to stay in Florida. Jack and I don't know what to do but we know we can't just pack up the car and head back to Maryland on schedule. When we talk about our options I insist we should just take each day as it comes and make the best decision we can as new information is presented to us. So for now that's what we intend to do. Nevertheless, I'm glad Dr. Vogel explains that Jack can get "a full cycle" of his chemotherapy here. I don't understand what a full cycle of chemo is yet, but Dr. Vogel says it's a 6-week cycle.

"What about the Dilantin? How long will I be on that?" Dilantin is Jack's anti-seizure medication.

I suddenly realize I must have a little more experience with seizures than I have with cancer. I've known children who have had seizure disorders. The base cause of the seizures must be treated, or in Jack's case, every tumor in his brain would have to be completely gone for him to be safe to go off the meds. I brace myself for Dr. Vogel's response.

"Mr. Shelton, you will have to take anti-seizure medication for the rest of your life."

The shock is evident on Jack's face. I wonder if this means the same thing to Jack as it does to me – that his brain will never be tumor free. I want to know what he's thinking but I also don't want to know. I don't ask.

Rather than address the bomb Dr. Vogel dropped, after she leaves our room Jack and I discuss our options for care and whether we should try to stay in Florida or get back to Maryland. When we moved to Maryland we knew we would spend a great deal of time in both states, so we enrolled in the Blue Cross and Blue Shield National Coverage Plan. Jack's care will be covered regardless of where we are as long as Jack's doctors are on the preferred provider list. Since Shands is a preferred provider we don't have to worry, all the doctors here will be part of the plan too.

We're more at home in Gainesville than we are in Maryland. And Kiley and Conrad are here. But because of Jack's work in the medical research lab in Maryland, he's acutely aware of the advanced treatments available to cancer patients at the University of Maryland Medical Center (UMMC). Jack feels he may get more cutting-edge care there. We're torn between our two homes and know eventually we will have to make a choice but we realize Jack isn't strong enough to travel. We decide to stay here for the time being.

"Since we have made this decision and we are staying here for at least the near future, we have to get your living will on record," I remind Jack.

"I know. The social worker has been hounding us daily about that."

Jack and I completed living wills in Maryland. They're on file at St. Agnes Hospital. "Should I call St. Agnes myself?" I suggest.

"No, I don't think so. I think I should reread and reconsider my previous decisions." There's trepidation in his voice. "These decisions look a lot different to me now than they did when I filled out the forms a few years ago before relatively minor surgery."

My hands shake as we talk about this. I can't manage to think about Jack being so sick he doesn't want medical intervention or that he may need to give me authority to make his medical decisions. I feel panic arising in me. I need to change the subject so Jack can't hear the anxiety in my voice.

I'm relieved when Dr. Pham and his medical oncology team, which includes Natalie Narain and Alexander Ruiz who are the intern and the resident, come to the room at 11:15 AM. For a few minutes I don't have to think about death and dying.

People come from all over the world to study here at Shands, bringing with them a richness to all aspects of life. This morning their diversity comforts me. Dr. Pham is Asian. Slight body, springy step, and quiet politeness confirm his heritage. Dr. Narain appears to be East Indian. Thick, dark wavy hair, richly olive skin, thin but with a strong physical presence that exudes knowledge and confidence. Dr. Ruiz is Cuban. He's handsome, with dark hair, sparkling eyes that reveal his playfulness, and a broad smile that brags beautiful white teeth.

Dr. Pham greets us, introducing himself and his team. His voice is gentle. "The pathology report has confirmed that your cancer is lung cancer that has spread to your brain."

Jack nods.

"I'm sorry to say, it is not curable," he continues.

Jack nods again. My stomach cramps.

"We can't resect the tumors. We will treat you with chemotherapy to try to control the spread of the disease, and hopefully to stop the tumors you have from continuing to grow."

I'm trying to follow everything Dr. Pham says. I watch him as I write down the words he speaks. The intern and resident are beside him, they look like a wall of white to me. A soft wall, but nevertheless a wall. My hands are shaking. Like the twisted tales we were told yesterday, the information about chemotherapy is different from what we were just told a few hours ago. Chemotherapies vary, I understand this part. They are generally administered every three weeks with successive treatments lasting as long as six to nine months. This doesn't match what Dr. Vogel said. It makes more sense to me to follow Dr. Pham's information than what we were told earlier since Dr. Vogel is a radiation oncologist, not a medical oncologist like Dr. Pham. And Dr. Pham is faculty while Dr. Vogel is not.

After a long pause, Jack asks, "What's the end game here, Doctor?"

"Mr. Shelton, we don't jump to the end game. We want you to focus on staying strong and fighting the disease. The radiation will target the tumors you have. Hopefully the chemotherapy will stop more from developing."

"You know my wife and I live in Baltimore. I work at UMB. Do you know anything about the medical centers in Baltimore?"

Although he's a small man, Dr. Pham is energetic and seems larger than life when he talks. "I know oncologists at Johns Hopkins and at the University of Maryland, Baltimore (UMB)."

The two men share names of people who work at UMB but find none they both know, which doesn't surprise me because Jack works in medical research and not patient care where he would be around more physicians. Jack likes it that way – too many people create too many distractions. He often describes himself as a "lab rat" and it's a good description. This conversation gives Jack time to build his confidence, to smile, to talk about his work. Sometime during this exchange, Dr. Pham started calling Jack Dr. Shelton instead of Mr. Shelton.

"I'm Mr. Shelton, Dr. Pham. It's my wife who is the doctor." Jack tries to clarify.

Dr. Pham smiles at Jack. I think we are missing a cultural cue or something because Dr. Pham continues as if he didn't understand Jack. "Dr. Shelton, I will be managing your care while you are here. I have ordered a CT of your pelvis, abdomen and skeletal survey because of the hip pain you experienced yesterday."

"I've spoken to my doctor in Baltimore about my hip but I am glad you are checking it out. Thank you."

"It's no problem. We need to be sure what is causing the pain."

I wonder why Dr. Weaver didn't order these tests. Jack was just in his office for his routine visit earlier this month. Jack gets regular blood tests and sees Dr. Weaver every three to four months because of his blood pressure. Dr. Weaver has Jack's blood pressure in control but what about the rest of his body? How could he have missed this cancer?

Dr. Pham continues, drawing me back to the conversation. "Dr. Shelton, you and your wife should discuss the options for treating the lesions in your brain." He continues to explain. Jack has the option for either whole brain radiation, which will kill micro lesions but also risks damaging short-term memory, or the targeted treatment mentioned earlier, which is called stereotactic radiosurgery.

"Dr. Shelton, first we will move you to the cancer ward. As soon as a bed is ready, you will be transported."

As Dr. Pham prepares to leave, he and Jack nod at each other in a gesture of respect. I feel calmness and quietness I have not felt from other interactions. I wonder if the feeling is disguised numbness, for we have just been told there "is no cure" in quite plain English.

Our discussion at noon with the two physicians from radiation oncology, Drs. Johnson and Armstrong, is the harshest yet. Again we're told that Jack's diagnosis is metastatic lung cancer and the medical oncologists will order chemotherapy.

As Dr. Johnson explains the radiosurgery, I can feel that Jack is not listening. I watch him. He can't continue comprehending, listening for hours on end. He can't absorb all this information. For the first time since his initial seizure, I wonder if Jack's mind is showing the effects of the tumors. Like he did yesterday, Jack keeps interrupting, asking question after question about his hand. When will it start working again? When can he get back to his lab?

Jack is also making repeated comments about the cyber knife, which is what the procedure is called at UMB. I can't even tell who the attending physician is – Johnson or Armstrong – because they are talking to Jack in turns, first one, then the other. Their approach is more like artillery shelling than a conversation, especially since it's obvious Jack isn't conversing with them but asking repeated, unanswered questions.

"Mr. Shelton, you need to focus on your cancer and the radio-surgery, not getting back to work."

Jack still either can't or won't accept this. He asks again, "Is it possible that I can get full use of my hand back? I need it for my work in the lab."

"Mr. Shelton, you are probably not going back to work," Dr. Johnson sounds exasperated. "You need to get your affairs in order."

I wonder if these words are part of the doctors' training. Can't they find a nicer way to say these things? Do we have to hear over and over again that Jack has no hope for a future? I feel very much like Jack and the two doctors are talking on three different tracks and no one is listening to anyone. The only way I can even stay in this room is to frantically write down everything Dr. Johnson tells us about the radiosurgery.

Radiosurgery will target all three brain lesions. First, an image will be ordered so that the surgery can hit the exact targets. We're not told where all three lesions are, but one is in Jack's left cerebral hemisphere. A pinpointed, high dose of radiation will be directed at each tumor.

The procedure has limited side effects, especially in compari-son to the whole brain radiation. The most common side effect is fatigue. Jack will need to go to "Monday afternoon clinic" to prepare for the Tuesday procedure, but there is no Monday clinic until January 9 because of the New Year's holiday and then the Gator Bowl.

I've always loved being a University of Florida Gator but when I hear that Jack's medical care is delayed for a football game, a slow boil starts in my brain. Jack's brain can just keep growing cancer while the universe turns its attention to a damn game. The only way I can turn off the flame that's heating my anger is to remind myself that it's only *our* world that has changed. Last year *we* were celebrating the New Year and watching the bowl games. Jack's cancer is *our* reality, not anyone else's.

Jack's radiosurgery will be done January 10. Then, after this radiosurgery, Jack will return every three months so the doctors can monitor his progress and determine if future treatments are necessary. The possible outcomes in three months are that Jack's lesions:

1. will be the same as they are now; or

2. will have shrunk and no new lesions have developed; or

3. will have grown, with new lesions appearing in his brain or elsewhere on his body. Radiosurgery is still possible if more lesions develop or we could opt for whole brain radiation.

My mind flashes to so many other images as these physicians speak. When you live in Gainesville your holidays are punctuated by Gator Football conquests. During the "Spurrier Era" Christmas was often second to football. Beer and chicken wings replaced eggnog and Christmas cookies. Orange and blue replaced red and green. During runs for either the SEC or National Championships, Gator paraphernalia dominates as many rows in the department stores as do holiday displays. Friends come together to assault the TV. We all feel warm and fulfilled when the Gators walk away with a win. Only five years ago when the UF Gators took on Ohio State for the National Championship, Jack, Conrad and I were partying in Conrad's friend Vince's back yard. Vince had moved his huge TV to the patio where a crowd of us enjoyed a bonfire and a smorgasbord of food while the Gators crushed the Buckeyes in their first ever meeting. It's another rematch this year. January 2 the teams will battle again. I wish fighting cancer was as perspicuous as fighting over a football.

These memories are intrusive but relieving. I constantly tell myself to stay here in the present and to listen to the information being shared.

I snap back to the present in time to hear Drs. Johnson and Armstrong confirm what Dr. Vogel said earlier – Jack will continue taking anti-seizure medication.

"What about the Decadron?" Jack asks. The Decadron is a

steroid he's taking for the swelling in his brain.

Drs. Johnson and Armstrong finally deliver news more relieving. "You will be tapered off as soon as possible." They continue, "Your chemo will not start until after your radiosurgery."

The natural blood/brain barrier we all have that prevents contaminants in the blood from crossing over into the brain require the timing of the treatments to be precise. Some chemotherapy is known not to cross the blood/brain barrier. This is important because when combining chemotherapy and radiation therapy, the goal is for there to be no cognitive side effects.

I can't absorb all this information, and if I can't, I don't think Jack can either. I desperately need to talk to Jack to find out how much he understands and can explain to me. All our lives together Jack has been there to translate technical scientific language into something understandable for me. But Johnson and Armstrong are barely out of the room long enough for me to start breathing again when Dr. Vogel comes back.

I look at the clock – it's still only 1 PM. Though it was only just a few minutes before 9 AM when the doctors started coming in and out of Jack's room, I feel like at least a whole day has passed. It's hard for me to comprehend that we're only through a half of our day. Jack and I have no time to talk. We have no time to process all that is happening, either as individuals or as a couple. Once again I'm so grateful to Carol. What do people do who don't write down all this information to reread later?

But wait. Taking notes doesn't just come from Carol. When we were kids my father was the champion of "taking notes." As a schoolgirl on a class field trip my father insisted I take a little notebook with me to the museum. Though I can't remember the name of the museum or what grade I was in, I do remember learning about flax and early American farm implements – better known to me as brooms. Because my fear of being laughed at by my classmates was not as strong as my fear of disappointing my father, I dug out the little notebook and hurriedly scribbled down a few words. In fifth grade our class went all the way from upstate to New York City. Again, my father insisted I "take notes" and provided yet another little notebook. On that trip I borrowed my brother Chuck's Kodak camera. I lost the camera and a souvenir bracelet I had bought for my mother, but my notes were safely tucked away in my pocket – again, successfully following my father's orders.

I'm on information overload and know I have the retention rate of a two-month-old puppy. And what's worse, we now learn that when they move us to the other floor Dr. Vogel won't be continuing Jack's care. There's a bed available in the cancer hospital. We'll be moved soon, but Dr. Vogel will stay working with patients in the "old building."

Drs. Narain and Ruiz will be Jack's doctors from now on. The last bit of care Dr. Vogel gives Jack is to confirm and explain scheduling the CT of Jack's chest, abdomen and pelvis. For this procedure, the technicians will deliver dye contrasts, and skeletal x-rays will be done first. Because of the dye contrasts, Jack will be put back on IVs to flush his kidneys. Dr. Vogel confirms the bone scan has been ordered, and finally, explains that because of the amount of fluids that will be given and taken from Jack in the coming days, a port will be put in to facilitate a better method than an IV.

The hospital has a transport crew. Whenever Jack needs to go to a test, one or two transport staff members come to take Jack. We keep the transport crew busy.

First they come to transport Jack for the CT scan. I know I need a minute alone to try to come to terms with what's happening to us. Whether or not he's capable of walking, Jack has to be in a wheelchair (or a bed) when being transported. Once he's situated in the wheelchair, I walk over, kiss his forehead, and say, "I'll be here when you get back."

As Jack is pushed out, I know I can't take another minute in this room. Realizing I have a limited number of minutes, I watch until Jack and the transport staff are loaded into the elevator and the door has closed. I push the button to call for the next elevator.

The sounds beep, the doors open, I step in. I'm grateful only three people are in the elevator with me. I pray there aren't too many stops on my way down.

I've been to Shands many times before, so when I get to the main floor I know exactly how to get to the exit. It seems to me that people are moving out of my way. They must feel my urgency as I jog through the halls toward the sliding glass doors.

Sitting on the edge of the wall in the flower garden, I call my sister Jeanne. I don't know why I dial Jeanne's number – but I also don't know why I called John when Jack had his seizure. Maybe it's because Jeanne's a Registered Nurse and I won't have to explain any details of Jack's illness. Maybe I need the mother/sister relationship Jeanne and I share. Jeanne is seven years my senior and often I've gone to her to talk my way through a problem or a decision. Jeanne listens, offers an opinion, but then lets me make my own decisions without making me feel like I have to follow her advice.

"Jeanne, do you have a minute? I just need to talk."

"Yes, of course. I'm so sorry Nancy. This must be awful for you and Jack."

"It is," I blubber. "Jeanne, they've told Jack he only has three to six months to live. It's horrible. Jeanne, Jack is so sick. I know he's dying right in front of my eyes." My face is wet from my tears and I can't control my sobs. My chest is jerking. My hands are shaking. I walk away from the public area hoping no one is watching me.

"I know honey. It's very hard. Jack's diagnosis is not good. And you know, Nancy, when the doctors say six months they really mean six weeks."

I cannot speak. No words come. I can't hear either. For me the phone call is over. I'm sure I respond in some way, but nothing registers. Whatever the reason was that I called Jeanne, it was not to hear this.

"I have to go back in Jeanne. They only took Jack for a CT scan and I need to get back in the hospital so I'm there when he gets back."

"Call me any time. Day or night. And Nancy, be strong. Jack needs you now more than he ever has before."

After hanging up the phone, I sit on another cement wall bordering a walkway. I don't know how I got to this place. There's construction around me somewhere. I can hear the heavy equipment. I turn my face towards the sun. The heat feels good on my skin. I lie down on the cement wall to soak up the warmth. I close my eyes and replay a day Jack and I spent on the river, hoping it will give me strength to stay positive when I get back in the building.

I can see us clearly. It's early in the morning. We are on the river in Jack's boat.

"Nancy, look," Jack whispers to me as he leans over the starboard side of the boat. I inch forward and spot two manatees.

"A mother and her calf." I whisper back. "How peaceful they are."

Jack steers the trolling motor to the right, and as we head into Kings Bay, we lose some of the clearness of the river and we don't see any more manatees.

Jack turns off the trolling motor, folds it into its mounting bracket, and starts the more powerful outboard.

We cruise out over the open water beyond the Manatee zone. Jack weaves our little boat in and out over the wakes other boats offer as airborne opportunities. I brace myself so my butt doesn't hit too hard as the boat slaps the water.

Jack's personality is like this environment – kind, warm, peaceful, beautiful. His muscular chest and arms excite my body, yet Jack's silent strength is his greatest measure of power.

Jack pulls back the throttle and lets the boat drift to a stop. We're by the wildlife preserve where the eagles nest. We sit in silence and enjoy each other's company without the necessity of exchanging words.

"You ready to head back?" Jack asks.

I force myself to agree. "I guess so."

It's this peace I need. I don't know how to find the quiet rest-fulness that was so abundant in my life just three days ago. I need the noiseless air, the stillness of life, the smell of open waters, the empty space that surrounds us when we are on the river. I need the noise in my head quieted.

I lift my body up off this wall that is radiating heat, taking the vision of our happiness with me as I walk back into the hospital.

The transport crew has come to take us to the cancer hospital. The walk is long. Jack's transport bed is stacked with our belongings. My feet hurt and I have trouble keeping pace with the two young people moving Jack – one pushing his bed feet first into spaces unknown to me, guided by the directing hand of his partner who seemingly sprints at the other end of the bed. Through corridors painted ugly drab colors. Through halls crowded with people. Into an elevator. A new world emerges, signaled by the ding of the opening doors and the flashing number eight above them. Down wide, warm-colored halls. The newness of the building both wel-comes and warns me. This space feels homier. Which feels much less temporary.

Rolling Jack into the new room is a routine event for everyone except Jack and me. Jack has never entered a room and moved directly to the center. He's a watcher – he stays to the side until he's comfortable. That matters not, his bed is positioned in the middle of the room with him in it, and everyone's attention is on him. I want to tell the people to slow down, to speak quietly, to give us a minute alone to enter this room our way. I can't. I move to the edges, voiceless, where Jack would be if he could.

The buzz of activity continues. Instructions are shared, a nurse introduces herself to Jack and someone writes his name on a white-board on the wall. Everyone is smiling. Except Jack. His eyes move from person to person. I can tell he's agitated but he shows no emo-tion to the nurse. He answers her questions quietly and respectfully.

We're barely in the room for 5 minutes when another crew

comes to take Jack to another test.

While Jack is gone, I start setting up our room, which is much bigger than most hospital rooms and has more of a hotel-type feeling than that of a hospital. There's a wall of windows with a picturesque view of Payne's Prairie. The building is clean and new. I unpack Jack's clothes and hang his shirt in the built-in closet and put my clothes and other odds and ends in the wood cabinets. I set out my books, Jack's magazines and both our computers on the window ledge. There's a small kitchen-like area with a sink and a counter. Clean, matching furniture includes a daybed/sofa, a comfortable chair with a footrest, and a traditional bed tray. A rather large private bathroom with a walk-in shower is just inside the entry door, out of sight from what's clearly designed to be "living space."

I sink down on the sofa. I lean my head back on the stiff padding and reach for a pillow to stuff behind my head. Just as I close my eyes, I hear a rapping on the room door.

As soon as Dr. Ashford, from radiology, introduces himself, I say, "Jack is still not back from the testing," hoping the doctor will exit to return later and give me time to rest.

"It won't hurt for me to explain everything to you first, and then come back and explain it again to Mr. Shelton. That will give you time to understand and ask questions before the procedure is done." Dr. Ashford's voice is patient, and I see the logic in his explanation.

I gather my note pad and pen, wearily ready to record more information.

The port will be surgically implanted in Jack's chest and used as an IV to give Jack fluids and to draw blood. Dr. Ashford explains that there are few complications involved in the procedure (only a small possibility of bleeding and/or infection and a smaller chance of bursting a blood vessel) and once in, there will be no more poking with needles and Jack will be much more comfortable.

"The nurses are very efficient but it won't hurt for you to be attentive to your husband's medications. It's important to make sure he doesn't get any blood thinners until the port is in place." Dr. Ashford assures me he'll return to explain everything to Jack, and leaves me alone.

I curl back up on the couch as I was before he arrived, but resting is impossible. I can only ponder the implications of what I just heard. A foreign object is going to be put in Jack's body. It will help Jack, I don't deny that, but still. Every time I run my hand across Jack's chest it will be there to remind me of the cancer trying to kill Jack.

By the time Jack gets back from testing, I'm so exhausted I rejoice that no more doctors come in the room for the remainder of the day. Instead of doctors, mental and physical exhaustion and hiccups are the invaders. Jack has a long history with hiccups and unfortunately, he's been hiccupping on and off since yesterday. The sudden eruption of sound as Jack's vocal cords snap shut because of involuntary spasms of the diaphragm muscle have become much more than the temporary annoyance that hiccups usually are for him. They are painful for Jack and cause mental anguish for me. They are a noisy, uncontrolled manifestation of the severity of Jack's disease.

All his life certain beverages have triggered hiccups for him – mostly Heineken or St. Pauli Girl beer but sometimes just Coke if he drinks more than one glass. Since he's had none of these beverages, we think one of the meds may be the cause. Jack's usual method of stopping them (holding his breath for a ten-count and slowly drinking ten gulps of water while exhaling) is only giving him temporary relief.

Since we actually have time alone together, Jack and I are finally able to talk. I tell him about the visit from Dr. Ashford, the port, and the need to monitor his medications. As I expected, Jack knows most of what I share. He has no emotional reaction to having a port implanted, only questions as to which one the doctors plan to use. He amazes me – he knows things about so many topics that I feel like he's a walking encyclopedia.

"How would you know about these medical ports? I've never even heard of them," I exclaim.

"I don't know, I just do." This is Jack – he just knows.

Kiley and Conrad arrive with a few things from home, including clean clothes, my mug, tea, and a boiling pot, my crochet bag and one of our recently delivered Netflix movies. They are showing a strong front but I know their pain is as deep as mine. Conrad spends a lot of time walking around. Like his father, he rarely stands still. He's managing to hold it together in front of Jack, as I mostly am able to do, but I know his sadness.

Conrad insists on driving me home so I can shower. He's right. I stink.

Kiley will stay with Jack while we're gone. The transport team is on its way to get Jack. He's scheduled for an MRI. Kiley promises to go with Jack and the transport team, to wait for the MRI to be done, and then walk back with him through the tunnel that runs under Archer Road and connects the various buildings. "Don't worry, Nancy, I'll write everything down if another doctor comes by. You go get cleaned up. A hot shower will feel good."

As soon as we pull out of the Shands' parking lot I lose control of myself. I'm moaning. My body shakes as I try to keep my grief in control. I lean forward in my seat and hug my knees and sob. My face is covered with tears. My nose stuffs up instantly.

Sitting back up, I utter the words, "I'm so sorry Conrad."

"Mom, what are you sorry about?" he protests.

Through my tears I try to explain. "I don't know. Your father and I have so many plans. We've been so happy. We just talked about how we were going to start putting money away to help you and Kiley buy a house. Now we won't be able to."

"Mom, that's the least of our troubles. You and Dad have already done so much for us. It's time to switch and let us help you."

I realize that's not really what I'm sorry about so I add, "I don't want your father to have cancer." My groans resume.

I hurry through my shower, pack as much as I can quickly realize I might need, and we head right back to the hospital. When Conrad and I walk back in the room, Kiley is helping Jack with his first hospital meal. She's cut up his chicken, opened his Coke (which he's really happy to have) and popped in a straw, and arranged everything on the meal tray so that Jack can start learning to eat using his left hand. We visit for another hour and when Kiley and Conrad head home, Jack and I do our best to hide. We want and need a private evening.

Our room is designed with an individual nurse's station just outside the door. A window allows the nurse full view of Jack's bed. There's a privacy curtain that almost completely closes us off to the station, but still allows a bit of a view for the nurses. With that view comes a small amount of light reflected from the hall. Determined to steal time alone with Jack, I pull the curtain closed as tightly as I can and wedge the visitor's chair against the curtain and the wall.

Jack shifts over and I climb up on the bed. We set up Jack's laptop and watch the movie *How Do You Know* and let Reese Witherspoon and Paul Rudd bring a measure of light comedy into our night.

The movie is perfect. It helps us escape. I feel the warmth of Jack's body next to mine, and there's no need to talk. Instead, we laugh.

After it's over, I reluctantly climb out of Jack's bed, move the visitor's chair so that the privacy curtain falls back in place, and retreat to my sofa bed on the other side of the room. In spite of the unavoidable hospital noise and light that invade the room and the unnatural physical distance between us, we both slide easily into sleep.

Friday, December 30

Jack can't walk without pain. We're scared. We're afraid the cancer is in his bones. We know the CT scan will show whether or not the cancer has spread to Jack's abdomen but I feel like I still need to speak to the doctors. All these days being swarmed with specialists have ended suddenly. It's a holiday weekend. Doctors are scarce and results are slower than normal.

Jack and I lived in Gainesville for twenty-five years and consider this our home, but we somehow forgot that the town's heart beats according to the university schedule, and on a Friday before a holiday weekend the action in the hospital will mirror the slow-moving, nearly empty streets outside.

Even though it hurts, Jack wants to walk as much as he can. Because of the repeated testing and the dye they use in the tests they have given Jack, he's hooked up to an IV saline solution to flush his kidneys. This morning when we went for our walk, we dragged along the pole with the hanging saline bag, but this afternoon the nurses explain they can disconnect Jack's IV so that we can move about more freely. As long as Jack doesn't stay disconnected for too long, we have the okay to take our walks without the IV pole. Since it's a slow day, we have time to become acclimated to our new temporary home. We're exploring "8 East" as it is called.

We find the "oven" for the hot towels and a huge moving rack of fresh towels and sheets that we're welcome to just help ourselves to when we need them. We snoop around the little kitchen. There's a refrigerator for patients and families so we don't have to completely rely on hospital meals. As long as we label everything with Jack's room number and the date, we can keep anything we want available to us.

Conrad was born here at Shands in 1978. It's so different now – it's a huge modern multi-complex of buildings dedicated to research and patient care. When Conrad was born it was imposing enough, and that was one reason we planned a home birth. Characteristic of the growing consciousness of the era, I had no intentions of succumbing to what I considered to be the dehumanizing ways in which women were treated during childbirth. Jack and I read everything we could about birth, we attended Lamaze classes, worked through a midwifery group, and prepared our home for Conrad's birth. Unfortunately, Conrad was as stubborn then as he is now and after three days of labor, we ended up at Shands anyway. Since midwifery was not legal at the time, our midwife was unable to come to the hospital with us, but she did drop us off at the ER. It was 4:30 AM, Monday, September 25, 1978. When we walked into the building, not a soul was in sight. Jack helped me to the row of seats and then hurried up and down the halls calling out, "Is anyone here? My wife is having a baby. Hello. HELLO." Finally, Jack found a custodian who located the admission staff, who processed me and moved me to the maternity ward. Conrad was born five hours later.

This cancer hospital is across the main road, Archer Road, but is connected by underground tunnels. The contrast between the old and new buildings is remarkable. Everything here is colorful and modern. There's a long common area along a vast wall of windows decorated with leather chairs and coffee tables. The artwork on the walls is all original, unduplicated photos – both inside and outside the rooms. Each picture was donated by a local person and is labeled with location and donor. Most of the pictures showcase the natural beauty of Florida. This touch alone makes us feel more at home than we have ever felt in a hospital. We even have a laundry room with two washing machines and two dryers and the nurses' station will give us laundry soap when we need it. Kiley and Conrad will be happy about this – they won't have to keep cycling dirty laundry and clean clothes back and forth.

Dr. Ruiz has come to visit twice today – once early this morning and then again this afternoon. There's a remarkable difference in how we feel about Jack's care when we have positive, comfortable interactions with the medical staff. I told Dr. Ruiz that his first name, Alexander, is one of my favorite names and he's demanding I call him Alexander at the same time he's insisting on calling me Dr. Shelton.

Kiley and Conrad have brought snacks from home and the area around the sink looks more and more like my own kitchen. My tea, mugs, plates and silverware I wash rather than return on Jack's tray are collecting so that I can serve our food from home whenever we want. Our room is just steps away from the little common kitchen and I'm able to get snacks and coffee for Jack as much as he needs or wants.

It's odd the role reversals I feel. At home Jack is the master of our coffee makers. We have "dueling coffee pots" as we call them because Jack drinks caffeinated coffee but I drink decaf. Every evening Jack washes and sets two coffee pots, one for each of us. And every morning I'm gifted by the rich aroma of his labor wafting up to the second floor, to our bedroom, to let me know it's time to start my day. But now it's me in the kitchen, running coffee through the commercial Bunn system and delivering the generic fresh brew to Jack.

The nurses in this building exude professional confidence and personal interest in Jack and me both. They are friendly and competent. At the hall's end there's a wall with framed pictures of the nursing staff and plaques that label their years of service at Shands. We call it the "Wall of Fame." It's impressive to see Jack is in the hands of people who have so much dedication and commitment to their profession and to this hospital. The nurses make me feel welcome, and though this is technically *Jack's room*, in all practicality it's *our room*. I have a bed, I'm welcome to use the shower, and the nurses seem to want me to monitor Jack's care. The staff delivers clean sheets, towels and socks for us both.

Jack's hiccups are cruel. They continue to haunt him and have become increasingly painful. The doctors have ordered medication to try to control them but we don't get the feeling there's a known course of action to treat hiccups. So far, whatever they have prescribed has not worked. Jack moved from the water trick to swallowing huge amounts of sugar – dry – to produce a gag reflex. That puts them on pause. But the only thing that stops them for more than ten minutes is for Jack to induce vomiting, which he has done several times since Wednesday night. We don't know what's causing the hiccups and we don't know how to get rid of them besides puking and I'm sure the medical staff would not want to know Jack is sticking his fingers down his throat when he really needs to keep as strong and healthy as possible to fight this cancer. I fear Jack will puke his guts raw but I can't make him stop and I can't tattle on him.

Gainesville has not been our permanent home for eight years and the number of close friends we have here has slowly dwindled. Jack and I have changed over the years. We gave up drinking alcohol and we value different things in our lives. I've kept in close touch with a few people, and of them Karen, Lisa and Danling are my closest local friends. I haven't called Karen or Lisa yet, but I have spoken to Danling. She was traveling all last week. She's home now and she's coming to visit us tonight. She's the first person besides Kiley and Conrad who isn't associated with Shands who I've interacted with since Jack's seizure.

It's late when Danling walks in the room. I can see from her face that she's overwhelmed with grief. We stay in the room and talk until Jack is tired and then Danling and I walk to the lounge area and sit looking out over Gainesville's night-lights. Tears come easily to us both. I tell Danling all that has happened these past four days and how afraid I am. She listens, quietly saying over and over, "Poor Jack." It feels good to be able to sit with my friend but before too much time passes, we part so that Danling can go home and I can return to our room to be with Jack.

I lie in bed, watching Jack from across the room, trying to figure out if I could make it through Mass tomorrow night. This year Christmas and New Year's, which are holy days in the Catholic tradition, both fall on Sunday so there's not an extra Mass. Almost a week ago Jack and I went to Midnight Mass together and if we weren't here in the hospital, I would go to church tomorrow afternoon. Christmas and New Year are the only two times I prefer going to Saturday rather than Sunday Mass. My family probably prejudiced me towards this because as a teen, my parents required us to attend New Year's Eve Mass before we were allowed to go out to celebrate.

I wonder if Jack will feel well enough for me to walk away from him, and whether or not I'll be able to leave the hospital if he does feel well. Will I just cry all the way through Mass? Would it be good for me to let all my tension out? I can't come to a decision. I fall asleep knowing that when I wake tomorrow I'll know whether or not I should go to church.

Saturday, December 31

I wake up feeling disconnected. For the past ninety-two hours I have slept on several different chairs and now a sofa bed. Jack has been pushed around, assigned and reassigned to "space" that is "his." This new environment is my new reality. It's distressing.

I realize I'm learning how to sleep with my head under the sheet. At home I need my face exposed, to breathe fresh air. But in this place I need my head covered so that I can stop the light from tricking me awake.

My body doesn't feel right. I don't have a headache exactly, but a dull tugging in the back of my neck. My stomach is heavy. Was I up too late last night? Am I afraid for the doctors to arrive? Have I missed the deadline for entering my semester grades?

Will Jack be able to stand up this morning?

As I lie here wondering what is wrong with me, Alexander shows up.

"Good Morning Mr. Shelton. Good Morning Dr. Shelton. How are my two favorite people this morning?"

"Aren't you in a good mood. You start work early – did rounds even start yet?" Jack smiles as he answers. Maybe this day won't be so bad.

"No, I just came by to see how your night was."

I never minded that Shands was a teaching hospital before but now I feel like Jack and I need consistent care over time. In a teaching hospital the attending physicians rotate according to a set calendar, which for short-term care is barely even noticeable but for us has meant a steady stream of new faces. And it's the last day of

December so the attending physician will change again tomorrow, but Alexander will still be here. Alexander is our hope for stability.

I feel more comfortable asking Alexander questions than I do asking the other doctors. He has a positive personality, smiles, and follows up when he says he will. He's youthful, and his youth projects optimism. He's also cautious about recommending medication for Jack's hiccups – he doesn't want to see Jack on psychotropic drugs if at all avoidable. This morning I want to ask Alexander about the swelling and droopiness in Jack's eye.

The change in Jack's left eye started a long time ago. I don't remember exactly when, but the first time I mentioned it to Jack we were in our family room getting ready to watch TV.

"Your eye is swollen. Are you getting another sty?"

"No. I thought I was but I'm not. I noticed that it's swollen too. I'm going to ask Dr. Weaver about it when I see him."

"Does it hurt?" I ask.

"No. Sometimes it's more swollen than at other times. But it doesn't hurt. I don't know what's causing it."

Now, after the seizure, the swelling has clearly intensified and Jack's eyelid droops worse than ever, I wonder if the earlier symptoms were missed signs of Jack's cancer. I've tried hard not to read anything on line about lung cancer since Jack was diagnosed because I want to ask Jack's doctors directly if we need to know something. But last night I was looking up the qualifications of the various doctors we have seen and there was a comment on one of the sites for Shands that stated a swollen eye can be a side effect of lung cancer.

"Alexander, what can you tell us about the swelling and droopiness in Jack's eye?"

"Why do you ask?" he queried.

"Jack's eye has been like that for a long time. I wonder if it wasn't a missed sign of his cancer."

"Well Dr. Shelton," Alexander smiles at me, "I don't know if the swelling he had before was caused by the tumors but I can tell you that if it was, there will be improvement after Jack's various treatments."

On the one hand this is a relief. On the other it only poses more doubt, more questions, more discontent. I don't understand how a man like Jack, under constant medical care by the same doctor for over five years, can have cancer go undetected as long as Jack's has gone. Jack's never hidden his history as a smoker from any of his physicians, was diagnosed with a peripheral artery disease that was potentially caused by smoking as far back as 2007, and yet was never screened for lung cancer? Not even given one routine lung x-ray?

After breakfast, Dr. Pham and his full team arrive. Finally, good news comes our way. There are no problems shown in Jack's hip scan. Jack and I exhale huge quantities of relief. Jack's radiosurgery will be done on January 10. There are still no pathology reports from the lab, but Dr. Pham explains the three possible results and how chemotherapy will be scheduled based on the results. Jack's chemotherapy regimen will be every twenty-one days but the duration of the chemo will be decided depending on the test results.

1. If Jack's cancer is small, "oat cell" carcinoma he will get three consecutive days of chemo, then wait three weeks, and get another three days of chemo.

2. If Jack has squamous cell carcinoma, he will have a one-day, four to five hour transfusion every three weeks.

3. If the cells are identified as adenocarcinoma, he will have a different drug than squamous cell but the regimen will be the same – one transfusion that lasts about four to five hours and is repeated every twenty-one days.

Jack is on the schedule for Tuesday when his port will be placed and his chemo will be started.

Kiley and Conrad are here this afternoon. We're laughing and enjoying each other as a family when Jack suggests we go for a walk. I dash to the nurse's station and request Jack's disconnection from the IV pump. A few minutes later Jack disappears into the bathroom and several minutes after that he emerges fully dressed. We three are shocked and so proud of him – he looks fantastic in his Gator tee shirt, jeans and Docksiders.

We walk to the elevator, head downstairs, cross the lobby and walk out into the fresh air and sunshine. I decide to stretch out on the bench in the sun while Jack, Kiley and Conrad take time alone walking along by the pond. The walkway extends around the water, which has a large fountain, through a small garden with flowers, benches and well-trimmed bushes. It's peaceful as I lie here in the sun. I had thought I might be able to leave Jack and go to Mass this morning but when I awoke, I had no desire to leave Jack's side. I don't need to be in a building full of people who don't really matter to me, mumbling words someone else decided are an appropriate way to seek what I need to be a good person. I need to be here, where I can care for and support Jack and collect information from the medical professionals as it is available. I need to be with my family. Before we walk back into the building I snap a photo of them. I want to remember this time exactly as it is – Jack, Kiley and Conrad. Together.

When we get back to our floor, Danling, her brother, and her sister-in-law are here delivering a dumpling dinner. Jack and I love Danling's cooking, especially her dumplings. Kiley and Conrad talk with us for a while and then head home. It's New Year's Eve tonight and before they leave they smile, promising to return later so that we can celebrate a little with them before they head downtown to meet friends at the bar. It feels so good to be social, to eat with friends, and to laugh.

Danling's brother is a doctor in China. He walks around the hospital to see how we Americans set up our facilities. He's extremely impressed, and I don't bother telling him that this floor is the best I've ever seen. It's okay to let him go back to China with an inflated vision of American health care.

Bill, Danling's partner, didn't visit with Danling and her brother but he sent an email that was difficult to read. Bill's father died without a will, which created a nightmare for Bill's mother. It has occurred to Bill that in Jack's and my situation, legal issues may be the furthest from our minds, so he sent a checklist of what we need. His words pierce me to the soul. I don't want to read this, but know I must. His advice is:

1. Make sure Jack has an up-to-date will and we understand how much money can be passed from Jack to me without paying inheritance tax.

2. Know that retirement, insurance, bank and savings accounts are passed to whoever is named on the beneficiary designation regardless of the will. Be sure we know who is named, and that there are records to be found.

3. A medical power of attorney (health care proxy) is needed for me to make medical decisions if Jack is unable to make them himself.

4. A living will is necessary, to state Jack's wish for care if prognosis and quality of life are questionable.

5. A durable power of attorney will allow me to act in Jack's place in all matters (except medical) if Jack becomes incapacitated.

I have to make several attempts to read Bill's email. I know Bill is right and I need to think of these things, but I can handle only a little bit at a time. Though I'm grateful for Bill's input I'm also angry that I'm forced to realize that cancer may very well render Jack "incapacitated" or, worse, kill him. The Shands social worker has been hounding us to get a living will on file and has delivered a pile of forms for me/us to read, but I just can't do it for the same reason that I feel anger now – I can't force myself to conceptualize more disaster or losing Jack.

Kiley and Conrad keep their promise and come back to visit us again. They're all decked out in their New Year's Eve hats and beads and are carrying bags, smiling as they approach us. Jack and I have never enjoyed going out on New Year's – we've always celebrated together, at home, not wanting to on the road on this night when so many people are driving under the influence. Though we would love to be *home* tonight, neither of us is envious of our kids in their pursuit of fun downtown.

We do, however, completely enjoy the hats, beads, and noise-makers they have brought us. The kids stay for about an hour, and when they leave Jack and I don our party regalia and go out walk-ing around the hospital, wishing everyone we see a "Happy New Year." We know we're an unusual couple on this floor where there's so much death and dying. So many patients and their families have perpetually sad faces, fear living in their eyes. Neither Jack nor I can succumb to that stance. We have to believe the New Year will bring us healing.

CHAPTER FOUR

The New Year

2012

Sunday, January 1

At the conclusion of every 60 seconds we live we have created another minute of our personal histories. Sometimes these minutes seemingly contribute little to ourselves, but other times we feel their impact on us in ways that make it impossible to live on as we were just moments before. These lived minutes continually add up and become our personal histories. Our histories form the individuals we are in the present and provide guidance and direction into our futures. As Jack and I move into the New Year, I know it's only our shared history that is giving us strength to face each moment with a positive attitude. Every minute is a struggle to be happy while it is also a gift that we're still together. Still communicating. Still hoping for more time together without dragging the weight of Jack's cancer with us.

Kiley and Conrad have been shooting video clips of Juno (and Gus) for Jack and me. Jack's dog is such an important part of his life. He talks about her every day and worries about her missing us. The hospital welcomes dogs as visitors, and Juno is coming to visit. But elevators scare Juno and at 145 pounds we can't just pick her up and carry her up eight flights of stairs to our room. When Kiley and Conrad arrive with our girl we go downstairs to them.

Jack and I have already taken one walk outside but it's a little later in the day and the sun is shining so brightly that the day feels much more promising. Jack's smile doesn't stop as Juno wags her huge body and leans into him for his loving touches.

Jack and I have owned a dog since 1982, usually more than one at a time. Until Juno, we only had Labrador Retrievers, or "labs" as they are most commonly called. It all started with Taffy. We wanted her to have a litter so that Conrad would experience caring for a puppy from birth. We kept two of Taffy's puppies, Cain and Abel. Cain's full name was "Raising Cain" and Abel's was "Abel to Please." They were perfectly named – Cain rarely behaved, Abel rarely misbehaved.

Eventually we gave Abel to my brother, Chuck. As Cain got older, we decided to get a chocolate lab puppy. By then Conrad was in high school. He insisted on naming her "Coke" finding great humor in having two dogs, "Coke" and "Cain." Jack said, "Just give her time, a good name for her will emerge." Since she was a strong swimmer and loved the beach, I named her "Coquina" for the amazingly gifted clam that buries itself in the sand and started calling her "Coquie." Jack and Conrad hated the name, and refused to use it. I had to have a name to give the vet, so I used "Coquie." Six months later we were watching our crazy puppy play with Cain and Jack said, "That's it. Her name is Coconut. She's a nut." We kept the spelling of "Coquie" but her name became "Coconut," and she was most often called "Nut."

We got Juno when Coconut was six years old. She taught Juno how to be a lab. Juno is a tennis ball retrieving, water-loving Mastiff. She'll curl up on my lap (if I let her) and is the most lovingly loyal animal we've ever had.

Conrad, Kiley, Jack and Juno head to the garden where they were yesterday and I retreat to the bench near the retention pond.

Jack needs time with Conrad, I need time in the sun.

I watch my little family together in the "Hope Garden" and wonder if I have any right to hope. I hate the garden's name. I don't want to find strength in hope – hope sets up expectations that can be easily unfulfilled. I want to find strength in science. Science is real, tangible, replicable research.

I rest my head back and close my eyes. But my brain won't rest. It fills with images of the new doctor we met earlier. It's the first of the year, the rotation has changed, and Dr. Pham will no longer be Jack's attending oncologist. Dr. Hyland is starting his rotation. Dr. Hyland has a soft, kind affect. He smiles more than the other doctors. He looks me in the eye when he speaks to me and he is patient when Jack takes time trying to express himself. His voice is clear, his speech moderately paced, and I can hear him with no trouble at all. As positive as I feel about him, he is still a new doctor, another unfamiliar person to step in and take control of Jack's care.

I wonder if these constant changes are one of the reasons Jack seemed nervous this morning. As bad as all this change, indecision, and lack of knowledge and direction are for me, they have to be worse for him. Besides the fact that Jack is a man of order, planning and careful decision-making, he's a scientist. And he's the one with cancer.

In spite of it all, Jack's pleasant demeanor holds steady. He asks the nurses and staff how they are every time they enter the room, says thank you to the nurses who bring his meds, the kitchen staff who deliver his meals, and the maintenance man who empties his trash. He makes jokes as a way of apologizing for the care he needs. I don't know how he does it.

Jack openly expresses his concern about his hand and his speech. Dr. Hyland assures Jack that his brain will continue to heal for three to six months and his strength and fine motor coordination, as well as his speech, will continue to improve. But is that enough? How can Jack's brain heal when it's full of tumors?

My mind floats to our future. Every hour is so touch and go that planning is darn near impossible. It would be easier if we just didn't plan, but took each minute as it comes. But how can you do that when each minute is so precious in terms of needing treatment? Dr. Hyland says they may *not* start the chemo Tuesday, January 2. If the lab reports don't come back, they won't know what chemotherapy to start. Dr. Narain had told us that the results will probably be in tomorrow but that remains to be seen.

My confusion is suffocating. It's not just the decisions about treatment here in the hospital, but what happens when we get out? We have to decide which medical oncologist Jack will see as an out-patient. Dr. Hyland suggests yet another name – Dr. Engle. He's a physician and lung cancer researcher. For some reason Dr. Hyland is under the impression that I had requested Dr. Norman. I clarify what I had said to Dr. Pham – only that I recognized Dr. Norman's name, not that I *requested* him. Many years ago Dr. Norman treated someone I knew, but I had no personal or professional relationship with him. I ask what physician Hyland thought was best for Jack and explain that we want the surgeon with the best background for Jack's cancer.

I had seen Dr. Pham this morning and he had asked me if we were still planning to see Dr. Norman. I said I didn't think so because Norman is a generalist. But Dr. Pham had said he was an excellent choice for Jack. I really believe each person on Jack's team is trying his or her best for Jack, but the angst surrounding every single sentence uttered drains every ounce of my energy.

The sun has warmed me well. I lift my head, open my eyes, and search for my family. I watch how relaxed Jack looks walking Juno around the little garden. Juno is wagging her tail and rubbing her head against Jack's leg as they walk. I've never known a man who loves his dog as much as Jack.

I walk over to the garden I hate called Hope. Jack and Juno take a few more laps and then Jack sits next to me on the bench. Conrad and Kiley are on the adjacent bench. I start to feel some of the tension escape my body. Juno flops her huge head on my lap. Jack chuckles and scratches her behind her ear.

"Nancy, why don't you and I ride back to the house together to take Juno home?" Kiley proposes.

I glance at Conrad. He's got one of those "Do it Mom" looks on his face. I realize he wants more time, time alone, with his father. "That's a good idea. I need to pick up different clothes and get the next book in my Vince Flynn series."

"Sounds good. Then this afternoon, we'll all watch the Denver game together." Jack's voice is cheerful. Conrad smiles at Jack.

I feel disoriented walking from the hospital to Kiley's SUV. I don't want to leave Jack. I don't want miles between us. I don't want to miss a minute with him. On the other hand, I know he needs time alone with Conrad and Conrad needs time with Jack. Besides being father and son, they are truly the best of friends.

Jack and Conrad are very much alike. Both southern gentlemen, they are men who don't yell in the house, don't curse at women, don't dash from task to task, and don't cause trouble with senseless talk about others. They have their flaws for sure, but overall they are thoughtful men who prefer to have pleasant conversations than to stir up tensions. When either man faces a problem, he analyzes it, decides a course of action, and proceeds towards a solution. During Conrad's teenage years he was sometimes disrespectful towards Jack. Since Jack's father died young, Jack's teenage years were father-less and he wasn't sure exactly how to handle the discontent Conrad was expressing. In typical Jack fashion, he quietly decided the best thing was to do nothing different. He was confident Conrad was capable of managing his own changing perceptions and that in the end, Conrad would come to the right decisions – right for Conrad and for those around him. Jack was right. And for the past decade Jack and Conrad have enjoyed the closest father/son partnership imaginable.

In the SUV with Kiley, I realize she has become the daughter I never had. We don't need to fill the air with chatter – we respect each other's trials, and will do as much for each other as we can do. I know I have drawn strength from her these past days and I know that she's selflessly giving me what I need.

I'm excited to see Tim Tebow play tonight. We are ordering wings from Wing Zone – complements of our friends Marcy and Matt – and though we will be here in the hospital, it will be nice to have a little football party in our room. When I married Jack I hated football. Jack wasn't a huge fan but football is an inescapable part of social life in Gainesville. Instead of fighting it, I joined the ranks of crazy football lovers. And I have to admit, being a Florida Gator has become a source of pride. I have three degrees from the University of Florida. I know it's a fabulous academic institution. But few people in the U.S. sit around on Saturday afternoons cheering highly effective teachers, astonishing research findings, and people who devote their life's work to improving the quality of life for others. Many people recognize and cheer athletics.

Jack and I belong to the Baltimore Gator Club. When we are in Maryland we meet with other Gators every game day. We watch a bit of NFL too, mostly to either support the Ravens or to follow the Gator players who have moved up. The Southeastern Conference (SEC) has become nationally recognized as one of the elite college conferences and our national championship years brought attention to individual players as well as the team. But all Gator fans know that many sports announcers seem to dislike the Gators. I can't help but think there are too many people who want to see Tim Tebow fail. First, because he's a Gator, second, because he's a Christian. The national controversy over whether or not Tebow can play at the NFL level is a welcomed conversation wedged between radiation and chemotherapy discussions.

Monday, January 2

Bright and early, 8:15 AM, Alexander enters with his usual smile. "Good morning Mr. Shelton. Good morning Dr. Shelton."

"Ah, there's the man. I saw pictures of you on the Internet at a party last night. You were all out of control."

"Mr. Shelton. You're teasing. I *was* at a party but no one was walking around with a camera."

"Well, I hope you aren't too hung over and can do your job today. I need you."

Jack only teases people he likes so I'm positive that he likes Alexander as much as I do.

The light conversation turns serious when I tell Alexander I'm extremely confused about the differing opinions between Drs. Pham and Hyland regarding Jack's outpatient doctor.

"You both have such a positive attitude you shouldn't worry about telling Dr. Hyland you're confused. He's a great guy and a great doctor – he won't steer you wrong. Talk to him."

After a pause, in a very personal voice, Jack asks, "What's the end game here?" Jack asks each of his doctors this, but I can tell from the tone of his voice, he's hoping Alexander might actually give him an answer.

"You shouldn't focus your thoughts in terms of the time you have to live but rather on fighting the cancer day by day. Keep taking walks. Keep doing as much as you can to enjoy each other. Keep being as positive as you've been. Just keep fighting." As young as Alexander is, he's able to speak softly and with great care in his voice, his eyes directly on Jack, his hand resting on Jack's shoulder.

Jack's fight needs to start with therapy. He'll be evaluated by the physical therapist (PT) and the occupational therapist (OT).

Before he leaves, Alexander warns us – the physicians won't be around much. It's a holiday. "If you need me tell the nurses' station and I'll come immediately. Since there are still no lab reports all we can do is wait."

The slow-moving holiday routine continues.

At 9:00 AM we meet Mary, the OT, who will set up an exercise program for Jack so that he can get back the use of his hand. Jack explains his speech difficulties to her – he can't pronounce the words he wants to pronounce. It takes him a long time to form some words, which are, for the most part, in his mind. Sometimes he can't recall a word but is able to substitute it with another, so he does. Mary will request a speech evaluation for Jack.

At 9:45 AM the PT, Hugo, comes to evaluate Jack. Jack's mobility is okay – he doesn't need PT, but Hugo recommends Jack start writing as much as he can as often as he can. Hugo explains to us that the hand-eye coordination and the cognitive stimulation will help Jack's brain heal from the seizure. He advises Jack to stay mobile and to walk as much as possible because cancer patients often lose a great deal of body strength. I wonder how Jack will respond to this advice. Since Jack's seizure he has not been able to read. Typically he would read a magazine a day when he's in the hospital but his stack of *Boating, Power and Motoryacht, Motorboat* and *Sport Fishing* rest on the window sill, untouched.

Another "white coat" is here in our room. I don't know the person's name or his area of specialization. He again explains the different cancer cells to us – small cell and squamous cell are treated with chemo, and non-small cell/not squamous means a mutation study is possible. Gratefully the person doesn't stay long.

In my mind I have come to call December 27 "Terrible Tuesday." Since that fateful day we have seen so many health care professionals that I can't count them all. And few of them seem to care that Jack is a microbiologist, one who has worked in genetic research for 30 years. Someone who is involved in research studies and who can better understand genetic mutations of the cells that cause cancer. Someone who just became a "subject" of his own professional career.

I'm tired of people talking. Almost a week has passed since Jack's seizure and he's had no treatment for his cancer – only relief from the damage the seizure caused and medical testing that so far has produced no useful information since the original diagnosis. I don't care that it's New Years, Sunday, a holiday. I want answers. I want action. Every day carries a fierce urgency that can't be calmed or fulfilled. Anxiety circulates in my body. These days with no treatment are creating an obsession in me that I control only by reading, writing and staring at Jack, silently, burning his image into my mind. It's as if the future does not exist – that I can look only ahead to the time and date of Jack's radiosurgery. Nothing exists after that. I can't see what might lie beyond – if anything does. At times I feel like Jack's seizure happened a lifetime ago and as bad as it was, it's gone now. It's over. Can't everyone just leave us alone and let us go home?

Jack's and my real suffering are not in the moments surrounding his seizure and diagnosis, but in these minutes when nothing is happening, our room is quiet, and there are no doctors, nurses or staff here. Just the emptiness that represents what our lives might be if the treatment doesn't work, or if it harms his brain. I have many questions that I can't speak, but I can write them down.

General questions to ask the team when we discuss treatment:

1. Does Jack need a power port?
2. Why did the neurosurgeons drop out of the discussion pertaining to Jack's treatment?
3. Why have we not seen a pulmonary oncologist?

Specific questions for selecting a doctor:

1. How many patients have you treated with Jack's disease?
2. What is your success rate with your patients with similar diagnosis and baseline health?
3. What homeopathic approaches do you combine with chemo and/or radiation? How do nutrition and exercise contribute to the treatment you recommend?

I start thinking about my sister Carol's impending visit. I need her here. She plans to arrive the day of Jack's radiosurgery. I wish she could come earlier because even though I know I'll manage, I really don't want to be alone.

Carol and I have had a strong sisterly bond throughout our lives. We played together as children, raised hell together as teenagers, and matured together as wives and mothers. Though we often depend on each other for emotional strength, we are also independent and have different ways of being that bring mutual respect. Whereas I would normally want to stay at Carol's house when I visit with her, she will prefer to stay at a hotel near the hospital and not at our home. I've been asking around to find out which is the best nearby hotel. All I can learn is where not to stay but Jack and I lived in Gainesville long enough to know the places to avoid so that's not much help.

Help. That's what I need. Where does one get the kind of help I need – the help that turns back the clock, that takes away Jack's cancer, that gives me back my life? Our lives.

Tuesday, January 3

Not only have I learned to sleep under a blanket to keep out the light, I've also learned to repeatedly start and stop my sleep. At 4 AM every morning the phlebotomist comes in to draw vials of blood. It is necessary – Jack's Dilantin levels must be constantly checked to make sure his dose is correct. The phlebotomists are efficient, in and out in a matter of minutes.

We wake for real at 7:00 AM. Jack immediately starts talking – he's on a mission. His colleagues in the lab, especially Jing, have been on his mind. I've been keeping in touch with his boss, Alan Shuldiner. Alan told me he needed to tell Nick about Jack's diagnosis because it affects the lab's overall ability to function.

I'm not surprised that Jack's colleagues need to know that he's in the hospital with an unknown future. Alan is set to start a new study with over a thousand samples that will be part of the study, all needing DNA sequencing. Together Jack and Jing coordinate that work. Jack and Jing work side-by-side in the lab, so much so that Jack calls Jing his "lab wife." Jack jokes that he says, "Yes ma'am" to me at home and "Yes ma'am" to Jing at work. Jack had a great relationship with Dr. Davis when he worked in his lab at UF, but there's something very special in his relationships with the people at UMB. Especially Jing.

I don't know Jing's perspective of Jack and their work, but I do know that Jack is an outstanding scientist. He's meticulously careful – as far as Jack is concerned, mistakes aren't acceptable. He approaches his work with a care that is truly rare. I know his colleagues need him.

Never the less, I asked Alan to please wait to tell anyone else. Jack wants to speak directly to Jing.

This morning I can't convince Jack to postpone this call any longer. I realize that besides Kiley and Conrad, Jack has only called his friend Pat. Nothing is going to stop him from speaking to Jing this morning, which becomes more and more obvious each moment.

At 7:42 Jack calls the lab. No answer. At 7:45 he tries again. This time he leaves a message. "Jing, this is Jack. Please call me on my cell phone when you get this message."

He's frustrated. "I want to talk to Jing before the doctors start their rounds. She's usually in the lab by now."

At 8:08 his cell phone rings. It's Jing. I can hear her scream from where I stand next to Jack's bed. "It's okay Jing. I'll be okay." But I'm sure she can't hear him because I can still hear her. The intensity of their relationship is fully exposed in this exchange. Jack continues to talk. "I WILL get back to work. I promise. I'll be okay."

I can only hear Jing cry and see Jack's tears.

The holiday is over for the medical staff, but with having had time off, they need time to catch up with all their patients. The morning lingers with little interaction with physicians.

Our first visit is from Dr. Ward and Nurse Tom. They are here to conduct a pre-op for Jack and to explain the procedure for surgically implanting the port for Jack's transfusions. Jack will get the "PowerPort" that can be used with dye because he'll need it for the testing that will continue to be a regular part of Jack's care.

They explain the process in detail. First they check Jack's vein, then shave his chest, insert the port, and put the needle in place. Jack can't shower for 48 hours, he's not to peel or flake off the glue they use for the procedure. From then on, when the needle is in place, we're to keep the port covered. When Jack is not in the hospital the needle is removed and the skin flap will cover the port so that Jack will have nothing to worry about – the port just becomes a part of his body.

Just after eleven o'clock Jack calls Jing back. These years that Jack has worked at the lab at UMB have been fabulous for him. He's highly respected and his colleagues truly like and care about him. He often asks me to bake breads and cookies so he can share something special. He talks about his days at work with a refreshing lightness – work isn't stressful for Jack. It's rewarding. He's proud of his knowledge, abilities, and what he contributes to the lab professionally and personally. That relationship has surfaced and I can see more than ever how important Jack's lab partners are to him.

Jack is able to tell Jing some details about his cancer diagnosis. She must have asked for our Florida address because I hear Jack giving her our street address instead of the mailing address. I'll need to send an email to make sure she has the correct information.

Before Jack hangs up I hear him promise Jing again that he will get back to work. Not a single doctor has given Jack the hope that he will be *able* to work again but he's obviously not listening to that part of the doctor/patient exchanges.

It feels uncharacteristic for me to just sit in the hospital all day, waiting for information, essentially closed off from the outside world. I normally spend my days between semesters reading, writing, interacting with friends, walking Juno, paying bills, cooking. When the semester is in session I teach evening literacy classes at the University of Maryland, Baltimore County (UMBC) and I spend school days at the Professional Development School where I've been the Professor in Residence for several years. When Jack isn't at work he reads the newspaper, plays with Juno, mows the lawn, reads his magazines, shops, and maintains our vehicles.

And especially now, when we're in Florida, it's odd to just sit. We're usually out in the boat, swimming with the manatees, visiting friends, going out to breakfast, lunch and/or dinner. But Jack is unable to read – when he's awake we "chat" or take walks. He naps frequently. When he's napping, I immerse myself in the Vince Flynn novels I had planned as my semester break reading. Little did I know the novels would keep me sane. They are the perfect books for the circumstances in which I now find myself. Mitch Rapp is fighting terrorism from abroad, Jack is fighting the terrorism of cancer. Mitch conquering the bad guy novel after novel lets me imagine Jack can be as successful.

We're just getting to know Dr. Hyland. His area of specialization is breast cancer research. He has a gentle way about him – another one of those southern guys. It's 1:50 PM when he comes to the room but he has so much information it's clear he's been working to get to know Jack's case. Though not 100% positive, Jack's cancer has been identified as Adenocarcinoma. I ask Dr. Hyland what this means in terms of how Jack's cancer may or may not advance, and Hyland explains that the lesions in the lung will respond faster at first if they are small cell, and that non-small cell are harder to get to shrink but they don't grow as quickly. So either way, there are advantages and disadvantages. Hyland is sending the cells for more genetic testing to check mutations that may also help to determine whether the treatment will be an oral chemo or an infusion.

There's no doubt that Hyland feels Dr. Engle is the best choice as Jack's outpatient medical oncologist. He has sent Jack's reports to Dr. Engle to review. This includes the CT, MRI and labs. Because Jack's cancer is atypical in terms of presentation, Hyland will coordinate with Engle to plan Jack's treatment. Hyland explains the decision-making process to us.

"The Lung Cancer Board will meet and decide what combined therapeutic treatment will be best for you, and which doctors are best to be on your team."

"When does this happen?" Jack asks.

"The tumor board meets every Friday, and this week, with all the specialists in the same room, they will discuss your case and come to some agreement as to how to proceed." However, Hyland wants us to be forewarned – often the treatment plan will change when more evidence becomes available.

When all the scientific information has been discussed, Hyland pauses, looks at Jack, then me, and back at Jack. Calmly he asks, "How are you holding up emotionally?"

Wow! I think. This man clearly has a different patient base than the other doctors. Hurray for breast cancer oncologists. Hurray for southern gentlemen.

Jack shrugs. "I'm okay as long as you all have a plan. My wife and I have decided we're in the 'Five Year Plan' and that means you need to be in it with us."

Dr. Hyland smiles and then explains how the outpatient services work. He wants Jack to be able to go home unless there's a reason for him to be in the hospital.

Jack, through hiccups as well as slurred and slow speech, says, "Being in the hospital is okay as long as I'm getting treated."

The two men talk about the brain's amazing capacity to repair itself, and Dr. Hyland again assures Jack that his speech will improve and that with OT, he can get back the use of his hand.

It was a long visit and when Dr. Hyland walks out, I move to Jack's bedside and put my hand on his, and just rest it there, hoping he's able to feel my love and to draw some measure of strength from our togetherness. After a few minutes, he looks up at me and I smile as I start one of our often-shared love exchanges. "Have I told you lately that I love you?"

"And I love you, too."

Dr. Hyland is back. He has already gotten a response from Dr. Engle, who has identified a mass protruding from Jack's kidney. Dr. Engle has ordered a new MRI to check the mass before discharging

Jack from the hospital.

Although we feel more tension building as we realize Jack has not been completely diagnosed, we're comfortable knowing that a good medical team is going to be caring for Jack. All three men, Hyland, Engle and Jack, are medical researchers – surely there is some sort of shared professional respect.

The Shands social worker comes to us daily requesting completed forms and we have put her off as long as possible. Jack and I use our time waiting for the test results to read through one of the legal documents we must face, his Durable Power of Attorney for Financial Management. His decision is clear and decisive. I'm his Attorney-in-Fact and Conrad is the Successor Attorney-in-Fact. What isn't clear is Jack's handwriting. He has to initial every section and sign the document. He's never had great handwriting but his signature today breaks my heart.

Jack can manage no more and I refuse to work through more legal documents. "Please come back tomorrow," I say as I take the paper from the bed tray and hand it to the social worker. She understands our grief and walks away without asking more questions.

Wednesday, January 4

Jack is and always has been a man of routines. Even here, in the Cancer Hospital, fighting for his life, he's worked us into a schedule. Each morning I get the newspaper and coffee for Jack and we start our day as much like we used to as possible. We no longer have control over when we eat and we plan our meals using the hospital menu instead of a grocery list, but we're trying to keep as much of our mealtime customs as we can.

Our shock in Jack's diagnosis is compounded by our confusion in how his cancer could have gone undiagnosed until it progressed to stage four. Jack is and has been under regular care and follows all his physicians' orders. He gets blood work and visits his internist every three months to check his blood pressure, cholesterol and general health. He was diagnosed with peripheral artery disease two years ago and he was put on a Mediterranean diet. A meat lover from way back, he even followed those orders to a T. It has been hard for him to eat beef *or* pork only once a month and chicken and fish just once a week. But he did it. And so did I.

Now that caution has been thrown to the wind. Bacon, sausage, and eggs fill Jack's breakfast plate, meat soups and sandwiches are part of every lunch, and meat is usually on the menu again at dinnertime. It's most important that Jack eat – he needs to keep his weight as stable as possible.

Since Jack is still having a hard time reading, I read the paper aloud and we talk about the news. We take walks as much as possible but we have to make sure we're not out of the room when the doctors make their rounds. As a precaution I've posted my cell phone number on the white board in Jack's room and I also tell the nurse on duty that we are leaving. Yesterday we got permission to take our walks outside. Jack is strong enough to go longer distances each day and the sunshine and fresh air help us stay positive.

It seems that the doctors make their rounds whether or not there's new information to share. At 8:15 AM Dr. Hyland comes in to let us know they still can't decide what chemo will be best until we know if the cancer is systemic. Dr. Hyland confirms that Jack's treatment will include chemo and radiation. The chemo will start as soon as possible after the lab reports come in. I think most people don't write down everything the doctors tell them so the repetition is probably necessary but for me it almost feels like assault and battery. Over and over we're told the same thing. As soon as I think this, another low punch comes in that is new and powerful – this time it's clarification that although there is a mass on Jack's kidney, they won't biopsy it. Apparently the doctors can tell whether or not the mass is cancer by determining if there's vascularity or not – if so it's cancer. I don't know what the hell vascularity is, but Jack explains that it means there's a blood flow. The doctors' "wait and see" approach allows me to put this discussion back to my mind's recesses, which is, at this moment, a good thing. I have too much information to figure out as it is.

After breakfast is finished, Jack and I decide to walk around the back part of the parking lot, loop around the hotel behind the hospital, and venture out to 13th Street. It feels odd to be walking on this stretch of road. We pass a seafood restaurant and true to form Jack stops for a menu. Walking away he announces, "If we have to stay at Shands much longer I'm going to send you out for a take-out dinner from this place." I suggest we just get permission to go out to dinner at the restaurant together since it's within walking distance.

After we get back from our walk, Dr. Hyland stops by again to let us know that the results for the tests on Jack's liver and kidney have come in – the liver is a cyst and the kidney is a hemorrhagic cyst. I'm too tired to ask the difference. I'm sure Jack knows already and at some point I'm going to sort out these terms. Cyst, tumor, mass, lesion… cyst, tumor, mass, lesion… cyst, tumor, mass, lesion… the words march across my mind like an army of evil soldiers.

Before the social worker's shift is over, we face the next legal document – Designation of Health Care Surrogate. This document is more difficult, but again, Jack isn't the least bit hesitant in his decision. If he's unable, I will make the decision to "withhold or withdraw life-prolonging procedures" or to "withhold or withdraw artificially provided sustenance and hydration," which would allow him to die.

Thursday, January 5

Jack and I have spent many hours discussing our options. Should we seek treatment at one of the Cancer Treatment Centers? Should we return to Baltimore for either Hopkins or UMB, where Jack works? Should we stay at Shands? Jack hates it up north in the big cities and he can't see going back right now as a viable option. He's at home here, for better or worse, and this is where he wants to be. He worked at UF for 23 years and this hospital is where Conrad was born. Jack trusts the environment and even though we've had our share of frustration with the doctors and rotations with this being a teaching hospital, Jack trusts the medical staff. That means a lot.

Jack is familiar with the UMMC because of his work at UMB. He respects it and knows he would get good care there, but Baltimore depresses him. He doesn't want to go up north yet. Philly, where there's a Cancer Treatment Center, would be even worse. It's farther north, I would be displaced, we don't know the city at all, and I can't stay with Jack at the Cancer Center like I can here at Shands.

We've decided Jack will start his chemo treatments here. I'm taking family leave from UMBC, which can be stretched for more than the semester. While I hold out hope, I fear the worst and deep down I'm afraid six months is all I will need. It's an absolutely awful feeling.

We're starting another day with Alexander's cheerful presence. He assures us that the radiosurgery is scheduled for January 10 and Jack's MRI on January 9 will confirm the exact target for the radiation. Jack expresses his concern to Alexander.

Before Terrible Tuesday Jack had no real trouble during an MRI. He never liked it, but he could bear it. He no longer can. "It freaks me out with the machine so close to my head." Jack speaks slowly, taking time to retrieve his words.

"Okay, I understand."

"I'm not sure you do. Or can. It makes me feel like I'm in a coffin."

"No, I can't quite understand that like you must. I'm sorry. I'll prescribe Ativan for you and any other drug necessary to help you through the procedure," he assures Jack.

The tumors in Jack's brain cause him to slur some of his words. He speaks slowly, haltingly. Some words he just can't say. He knows it's happening, so he stops in midsentence to find a new word. He hiccups constantly.

The respectful exchange between Jack and Alexander makes me think about the neurologists, who start every interaction with a mental acuity quiz. Interestingly, the questions don't seem to change. I guess if a patient can't remember, the repetition doesn't matter. But for Jack, with his intellect intact, the repetition is a bit insulting.

After establishing that Jack knows who he is, where he is, why he's in the hospital, the date, who I am, the questions become more difficult. "Mr. Shelton, can you tell me who is president?"

Jack knows what's coming. They don't just want to hear "Obama" so he gives them what he knows is next – "Obama, before him Bush, before him Clinton, then George H. W., Reagan, Carter. Is that enough or should I go to Ford and Nixon?"

The first time Jack answered this question, my mouth dropped. I couldn't rattle off these presidents in reverse order whether I was sick or well. I wonder what happens to people like me who don't store this kind of information – do we end up labeled neurologically impaired just because we're not walking historians?

Smart as he is, Jack's words come out slowly and are slightly distorted. Rather than speaking in sentences he speaks more in phrases. Halting phrases. With a lot of pausing between words.

But the fact that they come out shows that Jack's intellectual processing is unaffected. It also shows that Jack is aware of his communication difficulties. He apologizes for them and when he does, I feel his emotional pain. It hurts.

I've been drifting in my thoughts but am drawn back to the conversation when I hear Alexander talking about Jack's treatment plan. It turns out that the team has decided to do the radiosurgery before the chemotherapy. As hard as it is for Jack to talk, he's not giving up. "I'm concerned about the time lapsing before chemo is started."

"Too much chemo before radiation isn't good. The chemo sensitizes the body to the radiation." Alexander explains that the lung cancer is non-small cell so we don't need to hurry but we do need to move quickly for the brain treatment. And besides, Jack's medical team is still deciding which chemo will be the best to treat his specific cancer.

The team is considering a drug usually used with small cell for Jack. They've used it for other patients with non-small cell cancer with some positive results.

Alexander smiles as if he has a lollipop in his pocket he's going to whip out and present to Jack. "I have more news. Good news. You need to prepare for a van ride this morning. Since you're going to be discharged soon you need to be processed at the outpatient radiation clinic. This includes educating you both about the radiation therapy routine, touring the facility, and making the plastic cast they will use to keep you completely still during the radiation and protect the healthy parts of your body while targeting the radiation."

"All right. I'm up for that. Where is this clinic?" It seems odd to me that Jack and I have to ask a location of something here at Shands. We've been here for over a week. It's our new home away from home.

"It's a few blocks away from the Shands Medical Plaza," Alexander says.

"Here on Archer Road or is it on 13th Street?" Jack asks.

"Ahh. I forget that you worked here at UF. Sorry. It's on Archer Road." He continues, "I've already called for the van. They'll be here soon to pick you up."

Jack and I are trying to decide if it's good for Jack to be discharged. Every morning at 4:00 AM the blood draws continue. Every day the physicians change their plans. Sometimes even more than once a day. What will happen when we're no longer present in the hospital? How will we know if anyone is still paying attention to the latest test results, making sure Jack is receiving the best possible treatment? We're starting to realize that what *we* think doesn't matter, and we just have to make the best of whatever decisions are made.

The van ride is the first time Jack has been in a vehicle since the ambulance brought him to the hospital. The van is wide, fully equipped, and can transport more than one patient at a time.

The transport staff wheels Jack into one of the offices, where we will meet with the radiation oncologists. I feel so odd not being able to push Jack's wheelchair, to always have a transport person in charge of our direction, our schedule, our safety. Shands does a good job preparing the employees – everyone is friendly, efficient, and professional. Yet they are all strangers.

Suddenly, I'm stunned back to reality. The reality that used to exist outside this building. The one where I was a mother of a happy baseball player, and that happy kid had teammates I got to know really well because of all the hours we spent at the ball field. My life as a wife to the husband who used to man the grill, supplying the concession stand with burgers and hot dogs, while I took my spot on the bleachers with Coquie, who came to so many games she might have been confused as the team mascot. Standing before me in a white coat, holding a clipboard is Ray Glavine. I can't describe my shock but I know, all of a sudden, my past world and my current world have melded together and I recognize I'm living a completely different existence.

Ray Glavine, radiation oncologist, once outfielder on Conrad's high school baseball team, is part of Jack's team of physicians. Gratefully, Ray is personal, compassionate. But the amount of information is overwhelming. Once again I can only write everything down and hope that when I reread the notes I'll be able to comprehend all this information.

Jack's treatment is geared towards maintaining quality of life and hopefully extending it, but without Ray's kindness I know the coldness that I feel during this conversation will seep through my body and freeze me into motionlessness. As it is, I don't want to hear these words spoken – "We don't have a good cure for Mr. Shelton's cancer and there's a high probability that other spots will pop up even as the ones now present are being treated." Ray assures us that if new lesions develop in Jack's brain, whole brain radiation is still an option, as well as another round of radiation that targets new lesions elsewhere in his body.

I feel I'm drowning in the ice-cold water of a deep, dark sea. It is definite, they don't tell us why, just that it's the decision of the tumor board that they believe the best chance of stopping the growth of Jack's cancer is to proceed with nonconventional treatment – they are using a small cell approach even though Jack has non-small cell cancer. They don't deliver chemo and stereotactic brain radiation at the same time. The stereotactic surgery, or Radiosurgery is the *Linac Scalpel*, which was developed by two physicians at UF/Shands who are the doctors whose care Jack will be under. They will deliver the chemo and radiation to the lung at the same time.

Ray explains that lung chemo and radiation to the lung is not standard treatment, but standard treatment does not always work when treating gross lumps. They are using this nontraditional approach because the traditional treatment has been very disappointing for patients in Jack's situation. Jack's chemo will be administered every four weeks and will extend for six to twelve months. This will be coupled with the less aggressive three-week radiation treatment for Jack's lung lesion and not the seven-week treatment. I don't understand the decision to use the less aggressive radiation therapy and ask why Jack and I aren't included in any of the decision-making concerning treatment. I don't get a direct answer but an explanation of the risks involved in treatment, which is three-fold:

1. If all this doesn't work we have wasted three weeks of radiation treatment

2. The short term side effects include redness of skin, soreness in back, airway irritation, cough, shortness of breath, food pipe damage, difficulty swallowing, temporary tiredness. The degree to which the side effects damage the body is much greater with a seven-week treatment.

3. It is much more likely that major complications could arise with the longer treatment. Even with the three-week therapy, there's a five percent chance of pneumonia-like symptoms in the lung and a one percent chance of damage to the food pipe and spinal cord.

Because of the burns that can (and probably will) result from the daily radiation to Jack's lung, we need to make sure to use aloe lotion on Jack's back – but only after the radiation. The radiation therapy will end after three weeks and the doctors will follow up with a scan six to eight weeks after treatment's conclusion to determine how successful it has been.

Oh my God. I am so tired, and it's not even 9 AM. Here comes another doctor to join Ray. What do you know? It's Dr. Armstrong. The last time we met Dr. Armstrong she was with Dr. Johnson, when we were in the old Shands hospital building. Then the shock of Jack's diagnosis was fresh and raw, and the two women were trying to convince Jack he would not recover well enough to get back to work and that he needed to "get his affairs in order."

Ray immediately shares our personal history with Dr. Armstrong and slowly I notice a very different affect develop in her. Maybe it's my imagination, but I think she's softening, realizing we're just normal people, Ray's former classmate and teammate's parents, people who are just trying to hold on to some small measure of normalcy. Dr. Armstrong explains something that I'm sure is normal for her, but unsettling to us. She refers to the decision-making process for Jack's care as an *awkward situation* – one when the medical oncologist will make the final decision for Jack's care and the radiation oncologists will follow his recommendations. Another CT scan has been ordered and is scheduled for later today. For the first time, we learn that Jack's lymph node, the hilar lymph node in the center of his chest, is enlarged and the doctors suspect it's also cancerous. Comparatively, the tumor in Jack's lung is a fairly small mass and the treatment won't use a high dose of radiation. They will target Jack's lung and lymph node with this treatment but will use a low dose of radiation that is used for palliative care. A higher dose is used when the goal is to cure. "The goal for this treatment is to manage the cancer."

Manage the cancer! Are they insane? Who manages cancer? My mind is racing. My stomach locks in pain. I don't dare look at Jack because I'm afraid he'll see the fear and the anger in my face. I know

I have to stay as calm as possible. I focus on my breathing – slowly, deeply, in, out, in, out. With as calm a voice as I can muster I ask, "Why are we not trying to cure this cancer?" I'm trying not to alarm Jack but I'm on the verge of losing all energy. All composure.

The pain and tension twist and tighten when Dr. Armstrong responds. "The chance of it working is almost nil and we have to be concerned with balancing the cost with the benefit from an institutional perspective."

The cost benefit from an institutional perspective! Now I *know* they are insane. If Ray wasn't one of the doctors in this room and if Jack wasn't so sick I would start arguing with her. I don't know what to do. I don't know where to let my eyes travel. I feel totally defeated and have lost all confidence that we made the right decision in staying in Florida for Jack's treatment. We didn't have a choice but still, I wish somehow we could be anywhere but here, to hear anything but what I just heard, to know that Jack's colleagues back in Maryland were the ones making decisions for his care and not a doctor who has more concern for an *institution* than for my husband.

All I can think is *Just get me out of here.* Gratefully, Ray must have read my mind because he starts to explain that we need to tour the clinic and meet the LPN who will check us in when we arrive for Jack's therapy. I've never felt so grateful for the need to be "processed." I can't take another minute in this room with this woman. I wonder how she feels when she gets ready for work each morning, when she looks in the mirror and prepares to meet the day. I wonder if she's this cold to patients who have a better prognosis than Jack. I wonder if she has children, parents, brothers or sisters who may need a doctor to save their lives. I wonder how she would feel if her husband just got diagnosed with such a terrifying disease and she was the one who "had to get her affairs in order." We have to "stop by and see Dr. Armstrong every Thursday after Jack's treatment" and I wonder how I'll manage to do that with any measure of civility.

I'm detached listening to the nurse explain where we should

park, where to display the parking sticker, how to scan Jack's patient card, and details for Jack's diet and grooming. The nurse assures us that Jack can shower or bathe and eat normally. Normal – what exactly is normal? Honestly, I don't know and feel like I've never known what normal is. All this information being shared is recorded in a neat little packet that Kathy, the LPN, hands me. It's a good thing because I'm past the point where I can even take notes. I'm hoping somewhere in this packet they'll explain *normal* to me.

I want to drop from exhaustion. I'm mentally, physically and emotionally depleted. I have no more resources upon which to draw. Yet this day just keeps going on and on. It's like watching floodwater rise, inch by inch – you know major damage is about to occur but you can't stop it.

After we return from the Medical Plaza all I want to do is sleep. Or hide. Or get drunk even though I quit drinking over thirteen years ago. The hospital is in constant motion. Machines are beeping. Nurses are scurrying up and down the halls. The lunch carts are creeping from room to room. Before I can even make a cup of tea, Dr. Hyland is back in our room just checking on us and reminding us of possible side effects – Jack might cough up blood or display symptoms common to cold-like infections. It's exactly 1:00 PM. I've been awake for six hours but it feels like sixty.

Our respite from information and treatment lasts only an hour. At 2:00 PM Alexander is back and he's working hard to get Jack discharged. We're supplied with phone numbers, medication details, an appointment has been set up with Dr. Engle for January 18 at the Medical Plaza, and because of the possibility of another seizure, behavior restrictions are explained – no swimming, no driving, no ladders, no heavy machinery. *Are they really serious? Swimming! Heavy machinery! Forget them – Jack and I are finding the closest bulldozer and heading to the beach as soon as we bust out of here.*

The swinging door policy continues and Alexander is no more than gone when, finally, we meet Dr. Engle. I'm relieved to meet him and I can tell from Jack's attentiveness that he is too. I just wish I wasn't so tired. I haven't had time to process anything that has happened, to get questions organized, to prepare a coherent argument for more aggressive care. After all, Dr. Engle is the medical oncologist and therefore he's the one Dr. Armstrong has to defer to for all the decisions – the one who controls what Armstrong referred to as the *Awkward Situation*.

Dr. Engle is tall, thin, with dark hair and a pleasant quietness. We were already told that he's involved in research more than patient care, and he does seem like he's a man I should meet as one of Jack's colleagues instead of one of his doctors. He's formal, almost stiff, but listening to him I get the feeling he's intimate with the science of cancer and that's a good feeling. He explains, once again, that the plan is to treat Jack's brain with radiosurgery and his lung with aggressive chemo and radiation. He plans to coordinate the chest radiation and first round of chemo to be delivered simultaneous even though it's "unlikely to cure" Jack's cancer but will hopefully buy Jack time and control the possibility of new tumors growing. The chemo will be administered over a four-month period, with a dose every three weeks with continual blood work between treatments to monitor the side effects. Once again, this is different information from what we were told just hours ago by the radiation oncologists. *Yes,* I decide, *this is assault and battery. I'm so off balance I can't fight back.* Dr. Engle explains that he's going to be using a palliative dose. This is the second or third time I've heard that word, *palliative*, and I'm still not sure what it means.

Before Dr. Engle leaves he drops a bomb on us. "Hospice." That's all I hear in his garble of sounds. My hands start shaking. My stomach pains tighten. Dr. Engle is still making sounds but they mean nothing to me. His mouth is moving. I follow his gaze. He looks at me, then at Jack. Jack's lips are moving too but I don't hear him either. I don't know what it means medically to be in shock but I'm certain I qualify. I've stopped writing, stopped listening, stopped comprehending anything, and wish I could just stop breathing.

Dr. Engle exits the room and as normally as possible I tell Jack I have to go to the bathroom. I close the bathroom door and understand in a very different way what it means to spill my guts. I sit on the toilet as long as I dare, wash up, and return to Jack.

Jack asks me what I think about the suggestion to get Hospice Care. I say, "I don't know. What do you think?"

"I don't think I'm ready for that."

I've watched so many hokey movies and television shows where the teacher is "saved by the bell" and a touchy situation is diffused by the timely class change. I never think they are realistic – I'm a teacher and I've never been fortunate enough to be saved by the bell or any other routine part of school life. But today I'm saved by the routine part of hospital life, another interruption. Alexander walks in with Jack's discharge papers.

It's still going to take a little while to get out of here even though the papers are ready. Before we can leave the nurses need to train me. In my profession I refuse to use the word "training" but today that's exactly what I need. I don't want to learn what I need to do, I just need to be directed – give me the one-two-three step process to care for Jack and get his meds straight. I'll gladly be trained.

When Jack sees that I'm otherwise engaged getting directions for his home care, he picks up his cell phone. "Charlie, it's Jack. I just want to let you know that the doctors are letting me go home." I can't listen to Jack because I must get these directions down, but I couldn't be more proud of him. The fact that he took it upon himself to call my father is as revealing to me as Jing's screams were two days ago. Jack is loved. He knows it. And he loves back.

I sit next to Linda, Jack's nurse, who explains everything to me, step-by-step. Although she's reading from her set of papers, which will become mine, I can't just listen and believe I'll keep everything straight. So I take notes. Like I've been doing with all my notes since this nightmare started, I'm trying to color code these directions.

Monday January 9, 7 AM
MRI: check in at Far East of hospital MRI area.
Fill Ativan prescription to help Jack manage the MRI without panicking.

Monday January 9, 2:30 PM
Evaluation for Radiosurgery. Report to Neurosurgery Clinic which is on the 1ˢᵗ floor of main hospital, West of the Atrium in the outpatient wing, next to the coffee cart by the double doors.

Tuesday January 10, TBA *(we'll find out Monday during the evaluation)*
Radiosurgery.

Wednesday January 11, 10 AM
Appointment with Dr. Engle. Report to 2ⁿᵈ floor of the Adult Hemo and Oncology Clinic at Shands Medical Plaza.

Tuesday January 17, 11:30 AM
Report to Radiation Oncology Clinic; radiation will begin on Jack's chest; procedure will take about an hour.

Chemo MAY start the following Monday as they prefer to start radiation and chemo within a week of each other. Chemo will be administered at the infusion center.

Tuesday January 24, 3 PM
Follow-up appointment has been set up at the neurology clinic. Contact number is on official discharge papers.

Just because I've written all this down doesn't mean I feel confident that I'll be able to keep it straight.

The "Discharge Instructions" have summarized our last ten days in one short paragraph:

"Mr. Shelton you were admitted due to onset seizure. After an MRI it was found that lesions were found on three different areas of the brain one of them causing inflammation and edema. We also wanted to find a source of these lesions since you had no signs of infection. It was seen on imagining of the chest that there was a lung mass. Once stable with Anti-seizure medications and steroids to decrease edema as Neurology recommended we went forward to conduct CT-Guided biopsy. You were then transferred to Oncology

service. We then did subsequent imaging for staging to view other lesions. It was found that no lesions were seen other than benign lesions in the kidneys that were confirmed by an MRI. The Biopsy returned as Non-Small Cell Carcinoma with specific Bio Markers pending to direct treatment even more. During your stay you have increased strength and dexterity on your right side with normal labs and stable vitals. You are scheduled Jan. 10 for radiotactic surgery as you were informed earlier by Dr. Johnson. In regards to your chemo treatment Radiology Oncology will meet with your Primary Oncologist Dr. Engle in tumor board meeting tomorrow (1/6/12) to discuss your case. A lung coordinator will call you after she has the information that was decided to give you the schedule."

Linda and I go over these "instructions" and we both know that so much more has occurred, all of it necessary, all of it leading to the ability to write this short summary. All of it more emotional than either of us wants to discuss. Instead we focus on the reference to Jack's strength improving and the fact that *we are* checking out of the hospital.

It's late in the day before Jack is finally released. I have all the paperwork I need. Kiley and Conrad help us get our belongings packed. We're going home.

After two trips to their SUV, Kiley and Conrad return to Jack's room just as the transport team arrives. Hospital rules require Jack to be wheeled out, so he situates himself in the wheelchair. There are two more bags that need to be carried out. I put one on Jack's lap and the other on my shoulder.

As transport wheels Jack out of the room I see people lining the halls. Tears of joy and gratitude instantly fill my eyes.

I'm so proud of Jack and the way he handled himself as a patient. The professionals on 8 East are so kind and caring and Jack's interactions with them have been positive, thoughtful, and even friendly. Seeing everyone gathered is real evidence that Jack is not a number. Not just a patient. He's a living, loving person.

As Jack's wheelchair is pushed into the hall, the wonderful people of 8 East all start clapping for him. I realize that I am not alone in my hurt and we are not alone in our joy. This is a very happy moment.

Finally. We are back in our home. Conrad, Kiley, Jack and I together in the family room. Gus and Juno, the most farting-machine dogs I've ever known, never smelled so good. The trademark mastiff drool stains (we call them "slobber-gobbers") marking the walls are beautiful. A home-cooked meal. My own couch. My own bathroom.

"Dad, Kiley and I think we should turn Mom's study into a living room for you guys. What do you think?"

Conrad and Kiley clearly have figured out a way to make the house more accommodating for our long-term stay.

"It's a good idea son. We'll need our own space at times."

"It will be challenging to be together so much," Conrad chuckles, "but I think we'll manage okay."

Humor aside, we all know Jack wants to stay in Florida so we have to find a way to make it work. The front two rooms are two bedrooms, which currently are set up as a study and Jack's and my bedroom. Adjacent to the bedrooms is a front bathroom that is "ours" when we're here.

"We'll change the study and make it a second living room. We'll clean Gus's couch and move it into the room." Kiley explains.

Jack adds, "We can get another TV. I've been watching the new 3-D technology."

As I listen to this conversation, I realize that making these changes will give us the option to spend leisure time as couples rather than always being forced together as a foursome. Also, if Jack gets weaker, it will be smaller square footage for him to navigate.

I'm glad we have a plan for our living space here in Florida, but when I think about figuring out how to manage our house in

Baltimore I get weary.

Forget Baltimore. I'm going to enjoy the singular pleasure of sleeping beside Jack, in our bed, in our home.

CHAPTER 5

Home And Back

Friday, January 6

Our house is tucked way in the back of a private golf course community just north of Gainesville in the City of Alachua. It is the most peaceful place I've lived since my youthful days when I rented a little cottage on Gulf Way near the southern tip of St. Petersburg Beach, Florida. There I would wake to sea gulls screaming, and if my windows were open I might hear the waves meeting the sand on the beach across the street. Some 35 years later, it's a different kind of peace to awake to total silence but it's just as beautiful. Last night when I lay my head down on my pillow, I was next to Jack in the same bed, our bed, and not across the room from him. There were no machines around him, no beeps sneaking in through the cracks under the door, no LED lights flashing from medical equipment. Instead of inhaling the sterile smells of a clean hospital room, my nostrils were treated with the familiar house smells, complete with dog, dust and almost clean carpet. And this morning I'm snuggled next to Jack, feeling his warmth.

I lean up, my elbow bent, my head resting in my hand, and watch Jack sleeping. He starts to stir and looks over to me.

"Good Morning honey," I say. "How do you feel?"

"It is great to be home but I don't feel so good. My hip hurts quite a bit this morning."

The pain is similar to what Jack had experienced Wednesday, December 28 when he was in the hospital. At that time the physicians ordered a scan and reported back to us that there was no evidence of cancer. We figured the pain must be arthritis like Jack's internist in Baltimore suggested.

Jack gets up and tries moving around but he's moving slowly. The only meds that were prescribed and sent home with us were Dexamethasone, or Decadron, a steroid Jack will be on until the radiation oncologists decide the edema is safely reduced and the chance of a reoccurring seizure is diminished, and Dilantin, the anti-seizure medication. We have nothing more than over the counter remedies for pain because the only pain Jack has had is this hip pain, which was diagnosed as non-cancer related. We don't know what's safe for him to take and Jack doesn't want me to call his doctors. He wants to be home.

Conrad decides to wash his Jeep and though he's moving slowly, Jack joins him, out in the yard, in the sunshine. The two men talk while Conrad works. Knowing that Jack is in good hands with Conrad, I decide to go out in my car – I need to go to the bank, which is true, but more honestly, I just want to drive.

I don't plan to be gone long, but the freedom I feel is intoxicating, and I realize I need to see Karen. Karen and I have been friends since our sons played ball together as kids. We met when Conrad and Michael, Karen's son, were on opposing teams but before too long, Michael's father, Joe, invited Conrad to play on his team. Joe was one of the few youth coaches who ever really cared about protecting Conrad's arm and wouldn't let him pitch too long or throw too many balls. During that season Joe and Conrad developed one of the most respectful relationships Conrad has had with anyone outside of our family.

Later Conrad and Michael landed in the same high school and their friendship solidified. So did Karen's and mine. We worked one concession stand after another, from basketball to baseball seasons throughout four years of high school.

During their junior year, Karen and I even dared chaperone Spring Break at St. Augustine Beach for our sons and four of their friends. Conrad and Michael had reputations as hell-raisers with their teachers and other parents but Karen and I were delusional. We believed our boys could do no wrong. Our delusions were reinforced when the police came knocking on our condo door and the offending teens were not our own sons, but their friends. The ones with glowing reputations back in Gainesville.

It's Friday, though, and when I call I find that, as expected, Karen's not in her office so we can only connect via phone. I tell her as much as I can about Jack's cancer and promise to keep in touch, and I mean it. I know that I don't have time for friends, but I also know that I can't shut out the world or I'll be too weak to do what I need to do to help Jack.

After leaving the credit union, I drive across the parking lot to CVS. I buy a few supplies and head back home.

Jack's pain has not let up. By 4:00 PM he can no longer manage the pain and decides to lie down in bed with the heating pad on his hip. Gratefully, he falls asleep.

I'm worried and I don't know what to do to help Jack. For ten days we've had constant medical care and though I've often felt like I was tired of strangers controlling my life, I've had immediate access to medical intervention. It scares me to be alone.

"Conrad, how was Dad feeling this afternoon while I was out?"

"Not good Mom."

"Was it only his hip?"

"Yes. He wouldn't say anything but I know he hurt because he came in the house before I was finished washing the Jeep."

"Damn. I don't know what to do."

"Neither do I. This afternoon I hurried to finish so I could come inside with him."

"Thanks Conrad. I'm sorry I went out."

"It's okay. Now I'm going out. I want to get something for Dad."

I'm in the bedroom, sitting next to Jack on the bed, reading, when Conrad returns. He sticks his head in our room, smiles, sees Jack is still sleeping, and returns to the kitchen to help Kiley prepare dinner.

Jack wakes up just in time for dinner. He tries to get up out of bed but the pain is too great for him to stand.

"Well, it's a good thing I went to CVS for you." Conrad's grins, holding up a urinal.

"Damn son. I don't want that thing," Jack says, but he's smiling.

"You might not want it but you just might need it. Look what else I got for you old man."

"A reacher. I like that. I can pinch Mom with it if she misbehaves. And I like the cane too. Here. Help me see if I can get out of bed."

The pain courses through Jack's body. He tightens, unable to stand.

"Hmmm. I have an idea. Wait here Dad."

Conrad returns with the office chair. "Dad, this has wheels. Let me help you sit in it, and we'll get you out to the table for dinner." Jack is sitting on the edge of the bed. Conrad bends toward him, slips his arms under Jack's shoulders and around his back, half lifting Jack. The two pivot and Conrad lowers Jack into the office chair.

Conrad grabs one side of the chair, I grab the other, and we roll Jack out to the dining room table.

It's 6:00 PM when we say grace and start eating.

Jack's pain continues, even worsens. None of us knows quite what to say or do and the feelings in the room are stiff and tense.

We somehow make it through dinner, and roll Jack over to the family room.

By 7:30 PM Jack says, "Hey Kid, will you help me get to the room so I can go to bed. I want to put the heating pad back on my hip."

Conrad and I roll him back to our bedroom. Conrad reverses the same action he used to get Jack into the chair but this time, Jack screams out in pain. He is suffering. Trying hard to be quiet and unable to move, he's in worse shape than he has been since the seizure that started this horrible journey. I know we must get him back to the hospital.

"No, Nancy. I don't want to go back to the hospital."

"Jack, we don't even know what meds you can take. The pain is getting worse. We have to go. I'm going to call 911."

"No. Don't call."

Twin devils scramble my mind. One screaming, "Call, Nancy, you know you have to," while the other screams, "Listen to Jack, he's the one with cancer."

At 8:00 I dial 911. Jack no longer objects – he can't stand the pain any longer.

Conrad, Kiley and I leave the bedroom. The paramedics set up the stretcher next to our bed. When they start to lift Jack, a loud, terror-filled scream fills the house.

The drive back to the hospital is the opposite of a victory lap – I feel totally defeated.

The ER is a harrowing experience. Jack gets no pain meds. He finds one position for his leg that's better than any other, and I hold it in that position so that it doesn't move and the pain is at least bearable. For several hours I stand beside Jack holding his leg in place. I lose my own strength. My legs ache, my ankles are stiff, my heel spurs send shooting pains up my legs, my eyes are so tired my eyelids hurt, I'm afraid to move even an inch because every fidget causes Jack pain. Finally, the doctors give Jack morphine. He is being re-admitted.

The ER physician orders another bone scan.

Saturday, January 7

After 12 hours in the ER the transport team moves Jack back to 8 East. This time he's not in a wheelchair. He's transported in his bed. Jack wasn't even discharged long enough to lose his room, and we're right back in room 8206.

Because of the nurses and staff on 8 East, Jack and I both have a prevailing comfortable feeling even though we're here because Jack has been given a life sentence he's trying to get appealed. The wall of fame with their photos gives me a sense of security. As I pass their images I can't help but feel an overwhelming indebtedness to each of them for all they do for us. The nurses welcome Jack back with humor, teasing him so that his readmission isn't an embarrassing defeat. They seem to operate under the aegis of compassion while most of the physicians seem to be spokespersons of science. Of course we both love science – after all science has been Jack's life work. But our hearts need to be cared for as much as Jack's body.

The instructions supplied upon Jack's discharge obviously need serious revision. Yesterday I felt a bit of control reentering our lives and now here we are, once again, in a state of confusion.

At lunchtime Kiley and Conrad arrive with a container full of the ribs Conrad had grilled for dinner last night that we barely ate. "We knew you really couldn't enjoy the dinner last night, Dad, so we packed the leftovers for you."

"Thanks guys," Jack smiles.

They've also brought Jack chocolates. It would have been better to be able to share this meal at home but at least we can all be together here.

After lunch Jack naps. Having spent the night in unbearable

pain, he needs as much rest as he can get. Jack is terribly afraid to lose his mobility and for the first time, he's not keeping his cheerful attitude.

Bill, Danling's partner, sent another email. I can't believe how "on target" he is.

From: *Bill Lang*
To: *Nancy*
Subject: *Emotions*

Nancy, you and Jack are going through the toughest time in your lives, with unbearable physical and emotional pain now, and much more coming. Accept that all the rules of behavior have changed. Give yourselves permission to be who you are, and you must be, rather than what you think you "should" be. Whatever you are, whatever you are feeling at any moment, it is the right thing, it is good, and it is what MUST be.

You are going to feel what is happening is not right and not fair. And, you are right; it is neither right nor fair.

At times you are going to be incredibly angry at yourself, your partner, your family, the doctors, your friends. And ALL of these feelings are supremely right, and valid. Accept that you are going to go through incredibly intense changes in emotions in the course of a few minutes. You are not going crazy, you are doing what you must! It is OK!

You are going to be angry at yourselves for not being as strong as you thought you were. It will be only later that you realize that you were strong, and will have become even stronger. Your outlook on both life and death will change, as well as what is important. Pain makes us grow!

Don't judge yourselves for failing to live up to your unrealistic expectations of yourself and one another. The truth is these models were created by your ego. True strength can be found only when you are stripped of your ego, standing naked and without pride. And you will find the strength to go on anyway, because this is the only choice you have. Accept that you, stripped of your pride and ego, are beautiful and strong, much more so than when you are playing an ego role. You are real.

Give yourselves permission to lean on others, to expect "too much" of others. Those that truly love will understand, and give all that they can in return. There is no "you" and "me." There is only One, what we call "us," and we are going through this. Danling learned that lesson in her darkest hours with Xiaodi. She learned those that truly know how to love and help do so without the bullshit platitudes. Those that see this as OUR problem, well, forgive them for what they are, and love them anyway.

We will do our best to come when you want us and leave you alone when this is what you need. We cannot guess, you will have to tell us what you want, and with no apologies.

Thinking about you,
Bill

All I can say is that I'm already standing naked. And Jack is lying naked.

Jack's body is the constant focus of our lives, and conversations with the physicians are naturally dominated by facts and diagnoses. Dr. Narain tells us that there is, after all, a lesion on Jack's hip. It's cancer. A tumor at the head of his hipbone. Besides being in what he says is "the worst pain I've ever felt in my life," I can't know what Jack is thinking. I know how I feel. Overpowered. Scared. Angry. We went through this already and were told the pain was *not* cancer and now it is. Are we on a roller coaster? Or caught in some kind of human yo-yo that captured us and whips us up and down and all around at the end of someone's string? And why can't they get Jack on pain meds that don't wear out every two hours?

Dr. Narain is kind but I don't like what she's saying. Jack's pain will be managed with long acting morphine. The cancer is eroding into the bone, which is causing the pain. She assures us that radiation on the area will shrink the tumor, but even when they get the morphine dosed right to control the pain, Jack has to stay in bed until he gets the okay from Dr. Hyland to get up.

Thank God it's not long before Dr. Hyland walks in. He's angry and I'm glad. So is Jack. Dr. Hyland reviewed the reports that were sent to Dr. Pham after Jack's hip caused pain last Friday. The reports were misread. Jack should never have had to experience this episode of pain because the cancer has been in his hipbone all along. The tumor is perfectly situated to cause pain but not to cause other problems – it's sitting where the bone hits the socket. Dr. Hyland has ordered a higher dose of morphine so Jack doesn't have to request more every two hours.

Jack and I like Dr. Hyland. He has been more optimistic, more respectful of Jack's knowledge as a research scientist, and has compassion in his voice when he has to deliver bad news. And he's definitely delivering bad news as he tells us there's a possibility the bone involvement will change Jack's overall treatment plan. The cancer showing up in Jack's bone also impacts the chance of the chemotherapy being effective. He explains the concept of oligo-metastatic treatment, which, if I understand it correctly, is when cancer spreads from one spot to another. I don't really comprehend exactly what he's saying but I sure get the statistic he shares next – with each new spot the cancer spreads to, the chance for chemo to work is halved. So instead of relying on chemo, when a patient has oligometastatic treatment, the approach is more like "spot welding" where the oncologists fix only what is necessary to keep the body together. In other words, they will use radiation to zap the lung, lymph node, brain, and now hip.

Jack can't get out of bed until the tumor is treated with radiation because the pain at the bone stops his leg from moving the way it is supposed to move, which can cause other complications. Dr. Hyland will prescribe long-acting morphine to take the continu-ous edge off the pain and also make break-through pain treatment available. I ask what the "break-through pain treatment" is and Hyland responds that it will be the liquid morphine Jack has been getting. Together with the long-acting dose Jack should be more comfortable.

It seems a small measure of relief that the meds will be adjusted after the radiation works on the tumor. I have little experience with cancer but something in me fears morphine. In my mind first comes morphine, next comes death.

Dr. Hyland assures us that Jack will have future restrictions but he can be treated and get back to where he was before this episode. To begin with, he'll have to be careful making positional changes – when his joint's flat spot hits the bone, it will cause pain. This means walking will be fine, but Jack can do no lifting and must not stress his hip. Also, there's an increased possibility of arthritic changes developing over time.

The combination of morphine, pain, and Jack's bed-ridden status just gave this cancer power it didn't have 24 hours ago.

I am so angry tonight that I can't sleep. Jack's cancer should have been detected long before Terrible Tuesday. He sees his doctor in Baltimore three to four times a year, he goes for blood work before each visit, and he's asked about this hip pain.

And besides his hip pain, Jack has had incidences of involuntary kicking while he was sleeping that he also asked his doctor about, but no tests were ever run to find out what was wrong.

I don't understand any of this. If Jack's cancer had been detected earlier, he might have avoided the brain metastases (mets), the seizures, the loss of mobility. And I'm positive he would have avoided the pain he's having to endure now.

Why? Why? Why? How can lung cancer be so prevalent in this nation and yet go undetected so long that it has taken over Jack's body? Aren't there tests that should be run when a patient has symptoms like reoccurring hip pain and involuntary kicking?

And even this time, when cancer had already been confirmed in Jack's brain, lung, and lymph node, tests *were* run on his hip and the results were misread. How much pain and agony does

Jack have to go through before these people get it right? Doctors are not gods. They need to check and double check their work to make sure they have been as complete and thorough as possible. They need to realize that a seemingly simple mistake can rob their patients of life itself.

I am so angry I would like to cuss out the people who misread Jack's reports. I'd like to go to Dr. Weaver's office in Baltimore and tell him to take Jack's cancer and live it himself and give Jack back his life. I want to lose control, explode, rant and rave, throw books and files around some office somewhere.

But I can't. I have to stay calm. I have to act like Jack is not dying. I have to do anything and everything to help Jack. So I hold it in. I lie here in this pseudo bed, the blanket over my head, tears running down my cheeks, anger running through my skull, grateful that Jack is zonked out with morphine so I can cry without him knowing. I have never felt this helpless, this hopeless, this horrible in my whole life.

Sunday, January 8

Sundays are slow in the hospital, which gives me plenty of time to sit wordlessly worrying while watching Jack lay motionless in his bed. I turn to my book and read, then set the book aside, watch Jack for a while, and then read again. Then watch Jack again. I thank God I'm a reader and turn back to Mitch Rapp's heroic efforts to save the nation from terrorists.

Kiley and Conrad arrive after lunch. This is going to be a difficult visit. They are sitting together on the daybed/couch when we tell them that it's more cancer in Jack's hip bone. I see a visual change in Conrad's face. After a momentary stillness, he gets up and starts pacing. He's trying to be positive. We are all trying. But we've all hit the point well past how much bad news can be rationed our way.

Jack has no energy but much pain. He has had me ask the nurses for more morphine twice this morning.

At 1 PM another new face wearing a white coat comes into Jack's room. The information I'm able to capture from this visit all results from what feels like a question/answer session.

Amorosi: Hello Mr. Shelton. My name is Dr. Amorosi.

Me: Hi. I'm Jack's wife. Will you please spell your name for me?

Dr. Amorosi gives me a blank look.

Jack: My wife writes everything down. That's so we're able to remember everything. She's doing a good job.

Amorosi: Oh. Sure. A-M-O-R-O-S-I

Me: Thank you

Amorosi: Tomorrow the orthopedic surgeons will discuss Mr. Shelton's case.

Me: What time tomorrow?

Amorosi: In an early morning meeting

Me: What is your role in Jack's care?

Amorosi: Trauma service

He says something about "weekend consults" and then explains that the CT report the ER physicians ordered will be relayed to the orthopedic surgeon team. The team includes trauma and tumor specialists as well as oncologists. At 1:15 PM he starts to examine Jack, who is resisting all hip movement.

Amorosi: Are you in pain now?

Jack: Yes

Amorosi: Okay, Mr. Shelton. Just be careful and make sure and ask for pain medication if you need it.

The exam was short. He orders Jack to remain "non-weight bearing" and then makes his exit.

When Jack said I was writing everything down so we can remember, I wanted to blurt out, *That's not quite right. I'm writing everything down because I can't listen and don't want to hear this shit and writing is the only way I can even* try *to stay sane.* Writing is my primary way to cope with the overwhelming grief I feel. I can't think straight when my emotions are this raw. The amount of information that comes with cancer care is overpowering.

I'm living from one minute to the next just trying to make sense of the science and trying to savor the positive moments with my family. There's too much time to think when Jack is this bad and the medical staff is on a weekend schedule. I still haven't figured out how I'll manage to maintain our home (and Hei Mei, our cat) in Baltimore while taking care of Jack here in Florida, but it's more obvious with each passing moment that my presence in Baltimore anytime soon is highly unlikely.

Yesterday I sent an email to Katie (a former student at UMBC who agreed to visit and feed Hei Mei during the semester break) to ask if she will take Hei Mei as a foster cat until my life is straight. If Katie can help, Hei Mei will be okay. If not, I'll need someone who likes mean cats and can manage an indoor/outdoor cat for a while. I really wish Meghan, another former student who is now a close friend, didn't hate Hei Mei. But she does, and for good reason since Hei Mei occasionally bites and scratches people.

I also worry about our mail. I haven't made the house-watching kind of relationship with our new neighbors in Baltimore, since these past few months we have had a massive turn-around of residents in the townhouses adjacent to us. I've thought about for-warding our mail down here to Florida but many of the financial and most important documents I'll need in order to file our income taxes are marked "do not forward" and I'll really be messed up if I lose mail. There's a priority mail forwarding service available but I don't know if they forward "do not forward" items. I have to check on line but just haven't had a chance. If I can get the carriers to put the mail in the slot in the wood door (not the screen) instead of the mailbox, the mail would be protected from the weather and then someone could just send us weekly packages in a pre-paid priority mail envelope. I just don't know what's best.

I also have a house full of plants that need to be watered. When Hei Mei goes to foster care I'll need mouse traps all around. They will need to be checked every so often. I'm going to ask both Meghan and Morna to go by the house once a week just to check anything that might need attention.

As I think about how to solve my current problems, I realize that Morna's and my relationship *started* with me asking her for help. It was the summer of 2003. I had just earned my doctorate at UF and had accepted my first faculty position at Towson University. Towson is just north of Baltimore City and Jack and I would be moving with very little time to learn about the area. We had made a trip to Baltimore in June but it was a sellers' market and houses sold as soon as they were listed. We ended up explaining everything we needed (as well as what we didn't need – luxury) in a home to our realtor and signed a blank contract that she could fill in to use as soon as something suitable became available. Meanwhile, the Chair of the Elementary Education Department put me in touch with three faculty members who could act as mentors while I made the transition to Towson. Of the three, Morna was the only one who answered my emails. So when our realtor finally found a townhouse for us, I immediately contacted Morna and asked her to drive by and check out the neighborhood.

That was her first favor. And they didn't stop. Once we arrived, she welcomed us to Catonsville, delivering a housewarming gift with lunch. The adjustment for Jack and me was difficult but it became possible because of Morna and her husband, Len. They have become our family in Maryland.

But I can't ask Morna to solve all my problems. To begin with, I don't know what to do about the phone/TV/Internet services. Should I get them turned off for a time or just keep paying the bill? These are things I can't talk to Jack about, don't want to decide on my own, yet need to attend to soon. I'm not sure what decisions are best or if there are *best* decisions about *anything*.

I'm trying to read as much as I can while Jack naps because it's what little I have to help control my emotions. It's my escape. But I've set my book aside. I can't read. I'm livid. They need to start treating Jack and they need to get their reports read correctly the first time they do the tests so that this damn cancer doesn't have free range anymore.

The idea that they may not offer Jack the radiation treatment for his lung now that the cancer is in four areas is overwhelming. If that is what happens, I'm going to ask Jack's boss, Alan, to do what he can to get Jack better care. We've been promised the radiosurgery will still take place Tuesday and if something stops that, I think I may completely lose control.

I'm starting to feel my grief overpower my composure.

Monday, January 9

Dr. Amorosi wasn't kidding when he told us the orthopedic surgeons would discuss Jack's case early. At 5:30 AM another strange man wearing a white coat descends on us. This one is young. He has to be a resident – I don't even need to ask this time. I know that any information he's sharing will have to be confirmed, but he, Dr. Williams, explains the possible treatments for Jack's hip are surgery, radiation and medication, or any combination of the three. Dr. Williams suspects that multiple radiation treatments and medication (I presume he means chemo and pain meds) will be decided for Jack. He also lets us know that Drs. Adams and Oliver will be Jack's orthopedic surgeons of record.

Clearly the orthopedic group is efficient. Shortly after Dr. Williams leaves, another resident arrives. I've come to understand that the interns and residents have different levels of experience but I can't keep them straight. It's a good thing Jack and I are researchers and it's a good thing we like Shands, otherwise we would resent the number of people involved in Jack's care. As it is we find it difficult. When I talk to Jack about it he just says, "It's okay. We need good doctors and they need to learn. And this way we know we have people who are paying attention to me. Just keep writing it down and we'll keep it all straight." God, he has more patience than I. He's always been a tolerant person. I'm not so much that way.

This new doctor puts me at ease. He has a kind face and a great smile. His hair is the same color as Jack's and he's about the same size as Conrad. It's shocking to me that many of these physicians are just Conrad's age and they have Jack's life in their hands. But this guy, Dr. Spinella, is one I feel instantly confident about. I think he said he's specializing in orthopedic oncology – well, that's good.

"Spinella? How do you spell that?"

"Just call me Trey."

He spends a lot of time with us. I can tell Jack is comfortable with him when Jack responds at length to a question about his walking history. "I've had irritation walking from my car to my lab. I talked to my doctor in Baltimore about it, and he said I probably have arthritis. He hasn't done any tests recently though nor pre-scribed any medication. Now that we know this is cancer, what's the most appropriate treatment?" I notice Jack's speech is slowly improving. I like hearing him talk this much again.

"Mr. Shelton, chemotherapy presents risks for surgery. There's a high incidence of complications for chemo patients. It's major surgery that can involve bone cement with plates and can impede your functional capabilities. I'm in clinic today and won't be able to come by again until tomorrow, but we'll discuss this as soon as I can get here tomorrow morning."

It feels like the early days just after Jack's seizure. We're being bombarded with information, changing directions, and decisions other people are making. I need Conrad but he calls to let us know he has a cold, complete with a fever. He's not going to be able to come to the hospital until he's fever-free for three days. I realize but don't say anything – this means I'll be alone tomorrow morning when Jack has his radiosurgery.

By 9:30 AM the action has started. Someone comes in and

announces Jack needs to be transported to Radiation Oncology (Rad Onc). They load Jack with enough morphine that he can be transferred from his bed into a wheelchair but not so much that he's "loopy" as he calls it when the drugs affect his thinking.

Once at Rad Onc we're introduced to the head nurse, who starts sharing information with us so rapidly that I can't even record her name. "We're proceeding with the brain treatment. We need to get your pain in control and a week or so with the pain meds will help. Our second priority is your hip. We need a second treatment plan scan, but we know we can start your treatments tomorrow, Tuesday, or Wednesday at the latest. The treatment will continue for ten days. The treatments will be approximately ten minutes but the procedure will take about twenty. You can expect side effects."

She continues. "Side effects include skin reddening, but do not use any moisturizers before your treatment. The milder the products the better. You will experience irritation to the surrounding tissue. Also you will have urination and bowel movements more often and more urgently. However, if you have uncontrolled diarrhea or too frequent peeing we can use medications to control that."

As if these complications aren't enough, there's more. "Less than one or two percent of the patients experience additional, rare complications. These include permanent damage to the urinary tissue, permanent damage to the bowel, and the chance that the radiation doesn't work. If that's the case, you may have to have surgery to stabilize the damaged bone but this is not really a recommendation because it does not remove the tumor."

I have time for one thought while the nurse catches her breath. *This sounds abysmal!*

She finally finishes her "introduction to the radiation center" by confirming that Jack will have other treatments and we will be given more information about radiation and chemotherapy from Dr. Engle's team. Her final statement is, "You can expect the chemo to start 48 hours after the brain radiation."

She skillfully hands us over to the technicians who will make a body mold for Jack so that the radiation is directed at the exact spot it needs to be directed. I wait in a chair outside the room into which Jack disappears. It's cold. The wait is longer than I'd like. I'm shivering by the time Jack emerges.

Just before the tech starts pushing Jack's wheelchair we catch each other's eyes.

"Holy shit," I say.

"Yea" is his only response.

Our environments affect all of us physically, spiritually, emotionally and intellectually. Whether living in a home, a prison, a hospital, or any other space, the relationships we make within these spaces become our foundations for growth, change and learning. When Jack and I get back to 8 East, I know I need this environment every bit as much as Jack needs it. I need to learn more about Jack's disease, I need the nurses' support and knowledge, and I need the oncologists' expertize. I feel like we're back home when I step off the elevator.

Jack and I have come to call this place "The Blue Cross Hilton" because of the obvious effort the nurses and other staff members make to keep us comfortable. The environment is nowhere near as sterile as what I typically associate with "hospital."

The sheets, towels and blankets are hospital white, but Jack's bed is situated in front of a paneled wall that frames the bed similarly to a headboard. The outlets necessary for medical equipment are arranged in a row several feet above the bed so that unless I look up and away from Jack, they aren't even in my line of vision when he's sitting up in bed. His bed is flanked on either side by aesthetically pleasing cabinets, faux wood shelves, and a small clothes closet. The wall behind his bed is even painted deep green with an original, framed photograph of brightly blooming red geraniums. The floor is wood laminate, not ugly old linoleum or easy-to-bleach rubber flooring. Everything is clean.

We've missed lunch but we're immediately, without even asking, told the nurses have called down to get something delivered for Jack. "And Mrs. Shelton, can we get you something too?" Grateful, I ask for a small salad.

We barely have time to smell our food when transport appears in the door with a wheelchair and we're escorted down to neurosurgery. I have no jealousy of Jack being pushed in a wheelchair, but my heel spurs are so painful that I'm having a hard time keeping up.

Oh my God, this sounds like something out of a bad science fiction movie. That's all I can think as the doctors start explaining the procedure. My hands are shaking so badly I can barely write. My brain is numb.

This is all I can record:

"3-4 small screws
Novocain
metal ring
detailed CT scan
shoot hundreds of small beams of radiation
follow up with a scan every 3 months
85% chance of success
option of classic surgery if radiosurgery doesn't work
less than 2% complications that swelling could make tumors worse
can eat
can take meds."

One of the three doctors in the room hands me two prescriptions for Jack. One is for the radiation oncology clinic for Jack's hip treatments, and the other is for an "MRI – Head with contrast; S/P Radiosurgery for Brain Mets; due 4/2012." As I accept these two little pieces of paper I realize they hold the potential for my continued life with Jack. So much significance recorded on a prescription pad. I hurriedly shove the papers into my legal pad so Jack can't see my hands as they continue to tremble.

When I introduce myself to my students at the beginning of each semester, I typically say, "I'm a wife, a mother and a teacher."

These are intentional words. I chose them because I have always believed they define my most important roles and my most active relationships. As each semester develops into its own experience and I reveal more and more of myself, my roles as friend, sister and daughter also come into play. I've never been in a position to reevaluate this projected image, but today I realize I'm in that position.

All the days I've lived before this moment have made me who I am. I am who I am, not just because of my relationship with Jack and Conrad, but because of my identity as Nancy Lee Rankie, sister and daughter, who then became Nancy Rankie Shelton, wife and mother.

Since Jack's seizure I've almost insisted I don't need a visit from my siblings. I'm not sure why, but I've kept people at bay, not encouraging in-person visits, not allowing or making many phone calls, and emailing my family only sporadically. I generally call my mother, give her the information we're given from the medical staff, and ask her to share it with the rest of my family.

I know part of the reason I do this is because I can't handle distractions and still give the attention I need to give to Jack. Part of the reason is that I can't risk getting weak and breaking down in front of either Jack or Conrad. Part of the reason is that I don't want others to make suggestions about Jack's care, my role in his care, or what Conrad should or should not be doing. As the youngest of five siblings I'm more often given advice and directions than I'm asked for my opinion or to share my knowledge about any specific topic. The last thing I want is to be shoved into the "little sister" role or "the baby of the family."

I don't think my cautions have been unwarranted, but I also know that since Carol announced she's coming down to visit, I've felt a great sense of relief. I'm more emotionally exhausted and more physically tired than I've been since Terrible Tuesday. My feet hurt, I'm scared as hell about Jack's brain surgery, and I don't want to be alone. As Jack sleeps, I'm once again watching him, wondering what has happened to our lives. I cry, again, but only silently. I can't risk him waking, hearing my sobs, and seeing me sad. More than anything I need to be strong for him as he has been strong for me since our first date way back in 1977. And clearly, I need to be strong for myself.

CHAPTER SIX

Love, On A Normal Day

Jack and I often profess our love for each other. At various times the words hold different powers. One day it might mean we share a strong physical intimacy. Another day it might mean that one or both of us feel such peace and joy that it's only natural that we turn to each other in a sort of thanks – uttering those often over-used, barely original sayings like, "I love you lotses and lotses," a creative construction our son uttered in his preschool days but which continues to live on as part of our family grammar.

Other days we profess our love when we least mean it. The words are empty and hollow when our hearts are cold and tired.

But there has never been a time when I didn't want to "prove" my love to Jack. These past few weeks I've come to realize that love is not proven by logic, but by living in deep harmony with another person. Love is felt in strangely unexpected ways.

Images of our lives before Terrible Tuesday keep returning to me on my nights alone, awake long after Jack's snoring starts, after I've wet my bed with tears. One of my favorite stories we repeat to each other and laugh at came to be known as "The Mystery of the Upstairs Smell." Remembering these days when Jack and I perseverated over how our own selfish needs would be met in the midst of our chaotic lives helps me find peace, stops my tears, and welcomes sleep.

It was a cold Saturday morning in early December 2008. The mid-Atlantic sky was its usual dull gray. The sun had not shown itself for more twenty-four hour cycles than I cared to tally. I spent as much time inside as I could, working in our guest room where, if the sun dared peep out, it would burn through our windows and offer a temporary reprieve from a world of gloom.

After a cold, dreary, drawn-out week, Jack and I looked forward to going to the gym to work out. We always have energy together that we can't find as easily when we're living our separate work schedules.

This particular morning, I knew I had a few hours before we would leave the house, and during that time I was a woman on a mission. All week a powerful foul odor had permeated the upper floor of our townhouse. It kept getting worse, each day driving me to higher levels of irritation. In an attempt to find the source of the smell, I had closed off the rooms to determine where the smell was the strongest. I had opened the windows in the guest room and our bedroom, and with the doors to those rooms closed, I was able to eliminate them as the location of any foul odors. Nonetheless, I still had not found the cause of the smell.

"Jack, there's something stinking up here," I shouted from my office to our bedroom as Jack was dressing. "I've been trying to find what it is all week but I can't. Can you smell it?"

"No." A flat response. Well, what did I expect? He rarely thinks my concerns are worth his brain space.

"I searched all day yesterday for the source – something up here stinks. We have to find it."

The night before, after days of unsuccessful searching, I had gone to bed feeling defeated. But with only the bathroom and my office left, I knew I was close to solving the mystery of the upstairs smell.

I got down on my hands and knees to look under my desk.

Nothing there. I looked around the room. Too many piles. I'd have to clean out some of this junk. I put the garbage bin up on my office chair and started my attack. Within minutes two piles were tossed or shelved. Just as I started to feel successful, Jack yelled from the bedroom.

"Are you ready to go?" I heard the irritation in his voice and I wondered how two people who really do love each other can simultaneously be so grouchy to each other. "Why do you always think it has to be a dead mouse? Just because we killed one in the kitchen you think you have to smell one up here. Have we ever seen evidence of a mouse on the top floor?"

"Jack, I didn't say I smelled a dead mouse. I said, *Something up here stinks*. Please note, I said *something*. Why do you always have to think you know what I'm thinking instead of hear what I'm saying?"

"Well, we have to go. Please stop cleaning. We only have fifteen minutes before the Eye Clinic closes and I want to pick up my contact lenses on our way to the gym."

I looked down at the stacks of notebooks, the crate of student writing files, my paper cutter with all the scraps of sheared paper scattered beside it, and almost felt discouraged. I hoped my burst of energy wouldn't be depleted at the gym.

With my eyes lowered, I started to head out of the room. I saw another bag of books – so much to do. Then my eyes fell on a little blob of gray tucked up under the bag by the door, there it was.

"Ahhhhh. Jack," I yell, "I told you something stinks. And ha ha. There it is. A dead mouse."

I hate mice, alive or dead, but that morning I was so glad to solve the mystery of the upstairs smell, and I was so glad Jack had to eat his words, I almost laughed when I heard him gag as he bagged the bloated mass of gray fur.

What I wouldn't give for a week like this. The gray skies, the mice, the irritation in Jack's voice – none of it would matter. Even though I can look back and see those things wouldn't matter if I lived them tomorrow, the fact that Jack and I lived them in our yesterdays is more important.

Love wasn't then and isn't now something we can "prove" to each other in the ways we can verify scientific matters. We experience love in our belief that we can overcome hardships, calm discord, and support each other in times of need. Love is a feeling of oneness in thought, care, and compassion.

We approach love through a mysterious kind of faith, surrendering ourselves to unknown outcomes. Our love for each other is a matter of perception – we have no proof that emphatically verifies love is shared between each other.

I look over at Jack sleeping. Indeed, love is defined by experience, not science. It is not proven by logic but by living. I surrender myself to him, to whatever is to come.

CHAPTER 7

Treatment Begins

Tuesday, January 10

We're up early. The transport is here by 6 AM to take us through the tunnels under Archer Road to the Radiation Oncology Department (Rad Onc).

As we travel through these halls I feel like I'm in the hospital's bowels. It's a dreary place. And for me, it's scary. Though Jack is beside me in his wheelchair and the transport staff man is pushing him, I feel very alone. I wish Conrad didn't have a cold and could be with me. As we approach Rad Onc the empty halls are becoming sparsely populated. An open door here with human voices leaking out to the hall. A few people there outside another open door.

We turn another corner and pass a room packed with people sitting around a conference table. It looks like a large group of couples. Everyone is dressed in street clothes. Someone in a white coat is sitting at the head of the table farthest from the open door. I feel like I just saw something I wasn't supposed to see. Like I'm an alien and those people are humans.

The first thing the staff does is give Jack drugs. It's Ativan – he has to be rolled into another machine. Jack is becoming more and more petrified of these machines. I ask no questions because I don't want to increase either Jack's or my own anxiety. Mine is at the max and I'm sure Jack's is past that.

Next the staff shows Jack the metal ring they're going to attach to his head. I don't know what they are saying. My ears have closed. They're screwing the apparatus into Jack's head. I watch the skin in his forehead become more and more depressed. I can't believe this. They are breaking the skin. Jack has small leaks of blood.

The staff is kind. Their voices are smooth. I still can't hear them. Nothing registers except that they are screwing a metal open-like helmet on my husband's head.

Before I know it, they are rolling Jack away. He needs another scan. They need to make sure they direct the radiation beams into his tumors and not into the functioning parts of his brain.

I wait.

And wait.

They return, pushing Jack towards me. We're situated at the end of a dead-end hall, Jack in his wheelchair with this outer-space contraption screwed to his head and me speechless. Thoughtless. Spiritless.

Jack is being moved. I reach out to touch his arm. He can't move his head. I finally force myself to listen and am guided with Jack to the room where the stereotactic surgery will be done. The machine impresses Jack. He asks questions but they don't register with me. After a few exchanges between Jack and the Rad Onc nurse, she turns to me. "Okay, let me walk you out to the room where you can wait."

I turn to Jack. "I'll be here when you're finished." What a lame thing to say. But it's all I can come up with besides a much stronger, "I love you."

Someone is talking to me. She walks me to a room at the other end of the hall where I'm told I can wait for Jack. The room is beyond bleak. It's lined with old-fashioned hospital-like waiting room chairs. Fake leather. Ugly. Old. The room is frigid. I hesitate. The woman who has walked me out asks if she can get me anything.

"Yes, a blanket please."

"Sure. This chair pulls out into a bed. Would you like to lie down while you wait?"

"Yes, thank you. Would you mind bringing me a few blankets? I'm very cold."

The woman returns in a few minutes carrying sheets, a pillow and two blankets. I'm still huddling by the door. She walks past me into the room, opens the folding chair/bed, puts the sheet over it for me, positions the pillow and hands me the blankets.

The door closes. I set the two blankets down on the chair/bed and sit down. I open both blankets and arrange them so that I can cover my head and my feet. I situate them so that I can find them in the dark, get up and walk to the door, turn the light off, and carefully shuffle back to the chair/bed. I lie down and cover myself completely. "Scared" has shifted to "positively petrified." Hiding under the blankets I cry. I have to make it a fast cry because I can't have red eyes when Jack is finished. When I've let as much emotion go as I can, I switch from tears to Hail Marys. I stick with the Hail Marys until I'm only half conscious.

The procedure goes as planned and the transport is there to roll Jack back to our room. He's going in a bed and not a wheelchair. He said other than a headache from the screws they put in his head to hold the "ring" in place, he feels okay. He has three visible, swollen areas on his head with the same bandages I used to use when Conrad skinned his knees, but no other signs of having just been beamed with hundreds of rays of radiation to his brain.

We're back in 8206 and the nursing and transport staff (there are always two when a bed is rolled instead of a wheelchair) lift Jack from the transport bed into his bed when I see Jack's eyes flutter and his right hand raise about 12 inches and start trembling. Just as Jack's back hits his own bed I yell, "STOP! He's having a seizure!"

The transport staff step aside quickly. The nurse is on Jack's right side. I'm on the left. I hold his left hand – the one that's not seizing. "It's okay honey. I'm here. I know you can hear me. Don't worry, you'll be okay." *Damn. How can this be? He just came out of what was supposed to be a positive treatment for these damn tumors and now he's seizing again.*

The seizure stops. Jack is able to talk right away. He was conscious throughout the seizure. He could feel pain in his head, knew he couldn't control his hand, and, like the last time, tried to think his way out of the seizure.

The nurse writes down everything Jack says. She explains that the stereotactic surgery probably irritated Jack's tumor and he just needs time after the radiation for his brain to calm down. She reminds us that Jack's hip radiation is scheduled for this afternoon and she leaves to record the notes in Jack's file on the computer at the station just outside the room door.

Jack wants to rest. I hold his hand until he falls asleep. Then I move the chair next to his bed so I can keep my hand on Jack while I read. I want to feel him if he wakes up or if his body starts to tremble again. I look at the words on the page of my novel. I don't know what the words say but my eyes keep tracking from left to right, down each line. The details don't matter. Mitch Rapp is still trying to save the world from terrorists.

I hear the door creak. I look up. My brain signals my soul and I feel relief in every single muscle in my body. It is as if this horrible nightmare might in some way be calmed. I've always said that after Jack and Conrad, Carol is the closest person to me on the face of the earth. I feel that now – the emancipation from fear that comes only through the familiar touch of someone who knows your soul.

I had only seconds to feel this because while hugging Carol I see my brother John. My emotions switch to shock. John is here too? How's that? He doesn't even fly and no one told me he was coming. Oh my God. Jack's going to be so pleased to see both John *and* Carol.

It turns out that Carol had flown into Tampa this morning, rented a car, and drove up to Gainesville where she met with my brother, who had driven down from NY so he can visit Jack and me at the same time as Carol.

"Hi Jack. You don't look so good. I thought I better come down and make sure Nancy's treating you well." Carol knows Jack well. She knows he's not the sort of man who wants pity and sure doesn't want us to feel sorry for him.

"Yea, well, you know Nancy. She's still telling me what to do." Though Jack's smile is distorted, it is still obvious as he jokes with Carol.

"Oh you poor thing."

John approaches and I can tell he's out of his element. But he's smiling, putting his best face on and following Carol's lead. "Jack you had to go to these extremes just to get us down here? You could've just asked and we would've come without all this."

Conversation continues and I feel relieved that Jack's able to talk and visit. I've sometimes wondered if Jack is loved in the Rankie family, but seeing my sister and brother here is evidence of that love. In spite of it, though, I feel sad and stiff. I try to hide it but I don't know if I'm successful. If John or Carol feel my tension, they're kind enough to ignore it.

I want this visit to be in my home, where I can hand John a beer and Carol and I can walk in the yard and talk about things we don't want anyone to hear the way sisters do. I'm not "in" this conversation but I'm glad it's happening. I feel like I'm outside looking in on these three people. Jack, amazing as always, in a good mood even though he had his brain fried this morning and in a few hours will have his hip zapped.

Carol, knowing that softness is not part of her discourse with Jack, exclaiming, "This really sucks Jack, you were sure dealt a bad hand this time."

Jack smiles. His words are slow, and I miss what he says because

I notice how uncomfortable John is.

"Hi," John says to Linda, Jack's nurse. "You are Jack's nurse?"

"Yes. I'm on this shift." Linda smiles.

"I wonder what your background is. Are you a diploma nurse?"

Linda is comfortable and can even push back a little. "God, you are nosey."

"No, it's just that my wife is a nurse. And she tells me that she learned the most about what being a nurse was all about during her years in her diploma school program. There was more significant science and theory content in her degree programs. But the basic nursing content was strongest in the diploma program. Jack's my sister's husband – he's a good guy. I want the best for him."

"He's getting the best. He's a great patient and we're watching out for your sister too."

I watch this interaction and wonder what Linda is thinking. She's friendly, with an air of confidence. And she likes Jack. I know this interaction with Linda will help John feel more at ease as he gets to know how caring and competent all the nurses are – diploma or otherwise.

Before long 4:30 rolls around and it's time for Jack's hip radiation. We're back in the bowels of the hospital where the Rad Onc staff is ready to start the treatment. Jack is in the transport bed, John and Carol are near, and I feel less alone than I did this morning. Jack has rested and has more energy and is able to talk with John and Carol. All four of my siblings have been married and divorced but Jack has hung around. He always jokes that he is the longest-term "outlaw" in the Rankie family. "I'm the only original one left," he teases. Over the years, each of my siblings has created some sort of relationship with Jack, and he never perseverates on what might be "expected" of him in his role in the Rankie family as my husband. Instead, he has always found a way to make us smile and to engage in meaningful conversations. Generally, he gets along with everyone in my family.

Annie, the Rad Onc technician, explains everything that's going to happen next. They will bring Jack in the room, move him to the table with his special body mold in place, and then administer the radiation prescribed. Annie is friendly. She has a kind face and has a comforting maturity. As she starts to position Jack's bed so she can roll him into the room head first, I look at Jack to say goodbye and suddenly, once again, yell. "STOP. HE'S HAVING ANOTHER SEIZURE!"

I thrust the pad and pen I carry with me at Carol and quickly round the bed and get next to Jack. His eyelids are fluttering open and closed. There's a pause and Jack is still, but then his eyeballs start slamming from left to right without his head moving an inch. His left eye is more closed and his right eye is more swollen than it was before. His hand is not as raised or as trembling as it was this morning but it, too, is seizing.

When the seizure is over, Annie looks at me and says, "I don't think we will continue with the radiation this afternoon. Let's get Mr. Shelton back to his room to rest."

Back in the room Carol hands me back the pad and pen. I can't take them. "Can you keep taking notes for a while please?"

"Sure." I look at her and want to cry. I feel all my strength leaking out of my body. A doctor appears and interrupts my thoughts. I don't know him.

"Mr. Shelton, can you describe the seizure?" he asks Jack.

Jack's voice is more distorted than it was before. These seizures do something to his voice box, or his brain, or something. "I could feel pain in my head." He raises his left hand and says, "This hand is strong but my right hand is not. It's worse than it was before. I could push with my left hand and I did. I think I stopped the seizure by straining. I felt it start, stop and start again."

"Did you feel any facial distortion during the seizure like you did the first seizure?" I'm sure he's asking this because Jack's mouth is drawn down like a stroke victim much more then it was earlier today.

"No. And I don't like talking like this. I don't usually sound like this. I don't like it."

"The inflammation caused edema around your brain and your tumors are possibly back to the size they were before the radiation. I doubt the lesions are worse. I think these seizures are caused by the radiation." He explains that he will increase Jack's steroids as well as his Dilantin, the anti-seizure medication. "You had four lesions, two on the top and two on the bottom of your brain. I think the larger one caused most of your initial problems but maybe the smaller ones are making some problems too."

I'm confused. We were told there were three lesions. I don't know this doctor and I don't ask questions. Mixed messages are just part of life in this world.

The doctor confirms that Jack's radiation treatments for his hip will start tomorrow and continue for ten treatments that will be interrupted over the weekend. I don't understand this treatment plan. It seems that continuous radiation is most effective but we are going to start and stop for weekends? I thought medical staff worked seven days a week. I thought hospitals provided continuous care. I guess I thought wrong.

John and Carol have left for the night. They're staying at the Comfort Inn. I'm exhausted and ready for bed. This is a great room but my daybed that I make up every night is just too far away from Jack. Tonight instead of just getting my sheets and pillows out of the cabinet where I store them during the day, I start changing the furniture.

"What are you doing?" Jack asks.

"Getting closer to you. I can't sleep this far away. I need to be close enough to touch you so I'll wake up if you start seizing again."

"But are you supposed to move the furniture?"

"Jack when have you ever known me to care much about what

I'm *supposed* to do? I'm doing it. Period."

The daybed is heavy. I don't want to damage the floor. I lift one corner of the couch at a time and slide a washcloth under the leg. When I have all four legs on a cloth, I shove it slowly, pushing with my knees just a little at a time. I have the room half re-arranged when Jack's night nurse comes to check in. That's their routine and I should have paid attention to the time so that I wouldn't get caught in the act. Judy was just coming on duty – relieving Linda who had been with us all day.

"I don't think you're allowed to do that. According to regulations. Let me get your other nurse."

Judy returns a few moments later with Linda, who is featured on the "wall of fame." She's consistently provided competent, exemplary care for Jack. She looks directly at Judy, "I know the regulation is that we can't put anything near the bed that will obstruct access to Mr. Shelton. We can help Mrs. Shelton move this daybed so she can be close to her husband and so that she can quickly move the bed should there be an incident that requires emergency attention. Grab that side of the bed and help me arrange this please."

Linda asks me to step aside. "Judy, if you are questioned about this please just say I did it before my shift was over. I'll take full responsibility. Mrs. Shelton is caring for her husband better then we can and she's the one who knew before any of us that he was seizing. Twice. This is what is best for everyone."

When I climb into my bed, I reach my hand over to Jack and lay it gently on his arm. I can't believe I'm going to be able to spend the night touching my husband. What a gift.

Wednesday, January 11

"Good Morning Sheltons" jolts me out of my sleep. Trey's smiling face and his cheery movements top all previous crack of dawn visits to date. Before the sleep is even out of our eyes, Trey starts his explanations. "There are a number of possible treatments for your hip, Mr. Shelton. We have something called bisphosphonate therapy that is administered intravenously. The problem with that is a possible side effect of necrosis of the jaw. If you've had recent bone grafts we can't consider this. Also, we can use radiation on your hip to stop the tumor growth and therefore pain. Or we can use a combination of both."

"The bisphosphonate therapy is out." Jack responds. "I had a bone graft during dental surgery on December 5."

"No problem. We'll treat with radiation."

Trey and Jack continue light conversation during which Trey compliments Jack's attitude. "Staying positive will help your body heal."

"Trey, since you're in orthopedics, can I ask a question before you leave? Do you know if anyone can help me with my heel pain while I'm here with Jack?" I explain that I had started a series of cortisone shots in Baltimore that I had expected to continue. The pain in my feet is increasing exponentially. I need relief. Trey encourages me to go to the "Ortho Aftercare" clinic, gives me the hours and location, and insists I use his name when I check in so I'm escorted to treatment and don't have to wait and therefore be away from Jack too long.

Our usual morning routine continues as 8 East stirs to life. Coffee. Breakfast. Vitals. Before too long John and Carol are back. Jack immediately starts teasing John. "Well John, I guess I finally found a way to shut you up."

"Yes, Jack, you have. And I'd rather you didn't do it again."

"It was just a seizure John – nothing to be afraid of."

We have a chance to catch up on other family news before we're interrupted by transport. It's time for Jack's 10:30 radiation therapy (XRT). This time there's no drama and the treatment goes as expected.

We're back in the room by noon, when the physical therapist

comes in to work with Jack. John and Carol leave for lunch. I watch and listen to Hugo, the therapist, and Jack.

"I have a lesion on the top of my femur, or the roof of the acetabulum. What can we do for mobility?" Jack asks.

Hugo asks Jack's pain level.

"It's 5 when I'm resting or medicated. It was 9 during the seizure. It's 10 when my leg is moved."

"Can you move your leg on your own?"

"No."

"You are tensing your muscles when you feel pain. That's natural but it doesn't help your healing process. The XRT will improve your pain. When that happens we can work on teaching you to transfer into a wheelchair and eventually how to use the walker."

"How much weight bearing will I be able to achieve? And how much strength and movement can be restored?" Jack asks. His speech is slow and slurred but he manages to express himself.

"We will proceed with the goal of *maximum functional mobility.*"

That sounds like a non-answer to me. I watch while Hugo and Jack work through Jack's therapy.

"Mr. Shelton. Good Afternoon." Dr. Hyland notices that Jack and I aren't the only ones in the room. John and Carol are back from lunch. Jack immediately responds.

"My wife called in the troops. This is Nancy's sister and brother, Carol and John."

After the introductions have ended, Dr. Hyland hesitates just a second, and makes eye contact with Jack. "I have things to discuss with you. Do you want me to just go ahead or would you like your visitors to leave the room for a few minutes?"

"No, they're good. You can say anything you need."

"We've discovered that your Dilantin levels were sub therapeutic yesterday." Smiling, he continues. "You are a hyper-excreter."

Jack smiles too. "I'm not surprised. I metabolize many drugs more quickly than other people." Jack is very familiar with this since pharmacogenomics (how well people metabolize drugs) is exactly what Jack's research lab focuses on.

"We're going to keep checking your blood and monitoring your levels. There are many classes of anti-seizure medications and we will either use a different drug or higher levels of Dilantin. While Dilantin is an *oldie but goodie*, Keppra may be easier to manage your levels."

"It seems like every one of these seizures takes another limb. First my hand. Then my arm. Now my leg. How long is it going to take to get my body back?"

"Your recovery will last over several days. The radiation to your brain has caused inflammation. It will last for about 18-21 days and it has not peaked yet. But the brain is amazing and you can get all your movement back. We will get the medications at the levels we need because with each seizure, you increase the risk of having another. And if the seizures become widespread and generalized, they may take on different characteristics."

Dr. Hyland also discusses Jack's need for anti-anxiety medication. Since there have been so many MRIs and Jack has asked for the drug to get through the tests, Hyland wants Jack to know that Ativan is addictive with long-term use. Additionally, some of the other anti-anxiety drugs have been used to treat persistent hiccups. Jack makes it clear he wants no psychotropic drugs unless they are absolutely necessary. "I don't like feeling foggy. I just get high anxiety with the MRI. And I've always had white coat syndrome. This experience has not helped much with that."

People who suffer from white coat syndrome get elevated blood pressure when they're in the doctor's office or other medical care facilities. It's not surprising that Jack has it because an estimated one fifth of our population does, but it's more alarming for someone like

Jack than for others. Jack already has issues with his blood pressure. In fact, he's had hypertension since he was young. One night, back in those early days when Jack and I were just getting to know each other, we were sitting on Pass-A-Grille Beach watching the sunset, listening to the surf, amused by the pipers running with the waves when he revealed his condition.

"Nancy, I don't want to scare you but I need to show you a card I have in my wallet."

"Okay, I won't be scared of a card."

Sliding the card out of his billfold where other people keep cash, Jack showed me three names and emergency phone numbers. "I'm in a research study at the University. I have hypertension. I don't know whether the medicine I take is a placebo or the real thing so if I pass out or anything happens to me, you have to call one of these numbers."

I wasn't afraid then, but I am afraid now. For years Jack's blood pressure has been controlled but when he goes to the doctor he often has to stay in the office reading a *Boating* magazine until his body adjusts to his environment. Mentioning his hypertension to Dr. Hyland can only mean Jack is feeling a great deal of stress.

After Dr. Hyland leaves, Hugo, the PT, returns and works with Jack a bit. He works through several exercises that include lifting, chopping his food, straightening Jack's fingers, and increasing Jack's wrist and elbow motion. He encourages Jack to move his leg any way possible within his pain-free range. He reminds Jack to ask for pain meds and not to let pain creep back into his body. Before he leaves, he gives me a list of exercises (he calls it homework) for Jack's arm and hand that Jack needs to repeat up to three times a day.

At 2 PM Dr. Cao from the Department of Neurology makes his rounds. He explains in depth the initial seizure Jack had. It was a "Simple Partial Seizure" caused by his brain lesions. This diagnosis was based on the fact that only one side of Jack's body was "involved" and he did not lose consciousness. Dr. Cao explains further that one of the tumors in Jack's brain is close to the "motor strike region" and that has caused the facial droop and his right side weakness. The lesions and the edema contribute to the symptoms. The Decadron, a steroid, helps reduce the edema.

The constant repetition in what one doctor after another disseminates as privileged information can be annoying. I completely understand that Dr. Hyland is coordinating Jack's care and is the attending physician on 8 East. He's thorough, competent, and sensitive. Why Dr. Cao needs to confirm what Dr. Hyland told us earlier this afternoon (Jack is a hyper-excreter and metabolizes the Dilantin faster than other patients) is a mystery to me. Maybe it's because Shands is a teaching hospital.

Dr. Cao admits Jack's Dilantin level was low but denies the low levels contributed to Jack's second and third seizures – instead he claims the seizures were "break through seizures" caused by the radiation. Okay, we know all this. I feel like I have to listen to these facts with a constant job of probing for additional information. So I ask questions. I try to sort out the multiple mixed messages that are inevitable for anyone in our situation. I need escape from being repeatedly barraged with diagnoses when one quick shot would be so much more manageable. But neither Jack nor I have any power over either the frequency or the timing of our interactions with Jack's doctors. So with the opportunity in front of me, I push for answers.

"What are the exact desired levels for Jack?" I ask.

Dr. Cao does not look at me. Maybe he expects me to keep quiet and listen. I will not.

"And what are Jack's levels now?" I continue, making it obvious I will persist until I get answers.

"The desired level of Dilantin is between 1.5 and two, if Mr. Shelton's levels don't indicate the need, his dose can't be increased. Therefore, he will stay on the same dose of Dilantin and we will constantly monitor his level while he's an inpatient. If it starts trending down, we will increase the dose." Though he is answering my question, he refuses to look at me. His language shifts to address

Jack directly. "I hope the levels will be stable and we can discharge you Saturday."

I feel like I won a small battle of wills. I got a few tidbits of information.

We Rankies have the gift of gab. It's hard to get a word in edge-wise when two or more of us are together in a conversation. Sometimes it bothers me that we seem to talk more than we listen, but today I find it comforting. This afternoon when there are no doctors in the room, words flow quickly and easily between John, Jack and Carol. When I can, without feeling like I might upset Jack, I'm able to talk about my frustrations and this harrowing experience. It might seem like complaining, like I'm just finding fault, but I need to express my thoughts. Writing everything down is helpful but it's no substitute for human interaction and affirmation at a time like this.

Like the previous day, John and Carol stay late into the afternoon and then head to the hotel for the evening.

At 7:00 PM Alexander comes in for a nighttime check-in. He's so young and yet so sensitive to Jack's needs. And mine.

"I'm concerned about going home. I don't want to be pushed out of here before everything is set." Jack wants his position known before any decisions are made.

"We will monitor your levels for two days. The Dilantin levels need to be stable before you are discharged."

"The morphine seems to make my thinking fuzzy."

"Part of that might be postictal confusion that comes after seizures. But to be sure, we can take you off the morphine and try oxycodone. It's not as sedating. We can also take you off the muscle relaxant, Baclofen. The Ativan can also make you loopy. Reducing your dose to 1 mg will help."

"I don't know how stable my legs are and with the medication, it's hard to tell if it's my legs or the drugs."

"You need time to figure that out on your own. I'm hoping for in-patient XRT Thursday and Friday, and then discharge."

"I don't know. I don't want a repeat of the last discharge. I was back here before 24 hours passed."

"I understand. But there's no more irritation to your brain. More seizures are unlikely."

"What about my PT and OT? How does therapy continue as an outpatient? I want to get my body back."

"No need to worry, Mr. Shelton. Your physical therapy and occupational therapy can continue through outpatient services. The speech therapist who evaluated you has determined that your speech difficulties are neurological, not mechanical, and related to the upper motor neuron. You speech will continue to improve as the lesions in your brain reduce."

After Alexander leaves, Jack and I talk for a little while before Jack is ready to sleep. It's been a long day. I can tell Jack is afraid of being sent home before he's stabilized and I share his fear but can only reassure him that I think both Alexander and Hyland are sensitive enough to make sure going home is best, if indeed they send us back home. When Jack drifts off to sleep, my mind refuses to rest.

In my work as literacy professor and researcher terms like positionality, lived experience, and embodied ways of knowing are regularly part of my discourse. Tonight I'd have a hard time even defining these concepts but I know I'm living them. I know my positionality is shifting, my universe is changing. I'm living an experience that is crushing me. My typical ways of knowing aren't something I can tap into to manage my life. I'm not myself. I no longer know who *myself* is.

Because of my more aggressive, or as I prefer to call it, outgoing, personality, people who have observed Jack and me in public spaces draw the conclusion that I'm the one who "wears the pants" in our house. Jack's way of responding, "Yes dear" like a pussy-whipped husband and his aloof way of smiling as if he's just following orders is and always has been an act. Jack has been the strength in this relationship – he has been the constant, reliable, intellectual and emotionally sound partner who has centered us spiritually and emotionally for 33 years of marriage.

This cancer has completely disrupted the things about life that I knew to be true. Jack isn't just a cancer patient. All of a sudden he is my husband who has been handed a death sentence, and a very ugly one at that. I know deep in my heart that this cancer will kill Jack. I just don't know what the execution date will be. I won't let Jack know I feel this defeated and I'll keep verbalizing that I know he can be one of the outliers. And I'll agree with him every time – "We're in this for the 'Five Year Plan.'"

Jack has been my compass and I have been his. But his geo-magnetic field has always been stronger than mine. So many times in our years together I have waivered in purpose, direction, and desire. When that inevitably happens, Jack is the one who keeps me grounded. Our job histories are just one example. Jack has compromised higher salaries in the private sector for stability, health care and job security. He worked at his lab here at UF for 23 years. Since we moved to Maryland, Jack has been at UMB and he has no intentions of leaving. He loves his job. But I have already worked at two universities. Until my current job at UMBC I have never stayed in one position longer than three years. I get bored. The challenge in learning or accomplishing something dissipates and I have to move on.

Now, at UMBC, Jack has guided me to find ways to keep my job challenging and stimulating – something he has always done for himself. Suggesting I start new research projects embedded in my teaching, new collaborations with schools unlike any I have worked with before, and partnering with people whose research is very different from my own are just a few of the ways he has helped me find contentment.

Suddenly I don't have direction and I don't know how to make sense of the world. I don't have control. Jack doesn't have control. His body is broken. His mind, inseparable from his body, is equally as broken. These seizures just come in and take over. The tumors are unwelcomed guests we can't evict. Jack can't walk, has no use of his right hand, and sounds like a stranger when he speaks. When the orthopedic surgeons come in and ask him to move his left foot, he moves his right.

And then there are the hiccups. They erupt on the scene and send Jack's body into constant convulsions. They last for hours. Days. Now weeks. No drugs have helped for any length of time. We've been told the reason cancer patients sometimes have hiccups is scientifically unknown. We know of no research being done to find a cause or a cure. Something as small as a hiccup has exploded to become a terrorizing force every bit as frightening as Al Qaeda forces storming the hospital lobby.

Thursday, January 12, Early Morning

"Good Morning Sheltons." Usually Trey's cheerful greeting filling the room startles me out of sleep but not this morning – I've been awake for at least an hour. I have a million questions that jarred me out of sleep and I needed to hurriedly write them down before they leaked out of my brain.

"Good Morning Trey. I'm ready for you this morning."

"Great. What can I help you with?"

"Question Number One – What does non-weight bearing mean? Please tell me exactly in terms of standing, sitting, walking and bathing. What can and can't be done?"

"For Mr. Shelton, you should put only about forty percent of your weight on your hip at any given time in any given position. You can put your foot down, but be very careful shifting your weight."

"Thanks. Question Number Two – What are Jack's expectation for mobility and weight bearing as a result of two to three days of XRT?"

Trey speaks with confidence and compassion. "We'll follow the

XRT up with x-rays. His level of pain will determine Mr. Shelton's movement. His case will be presented tomorrow morning at the Sarcoma/Carcinoma Board meeting."

It's becoming more and more obvious to me that we have little to no decision-making power when it comes to Jack's care. Instead of fretting, I force myself to visualize a positive report from tomorrow's meeting.

I move to the chair in the corner of the room, slump down, close my eyes, not even listening to Trey and Jack, and let numbness take over.

Conrad's fever is gone and he's here early this morning. Before he got sick he was at the hospital every day but we haven't wanted him here for long periods of time. We don't want him to hang around the hospital, to be here for all of Jack's tests (and results), or for every meal. We want him to come and go in a more natural way. We want him to be here with purpose, to do what he needs to do, and then to go home and come back when he needs to (or we need him to).

Conrad is like his father – he gets along with all the Rankies, and he manages to smile and let comments my family make that irk me just fade into the atmosphere. But I have no time to help Conrad cope with Jack's cancer, and I'm glad he's well enough to come spend time with John and Carol. He needs my family. His family.

More so than any other day since Jack's first seizure, a lot of energy is being expended in this room. John and Carol keep lively conversation going amongst everyone, including the medical staff who are in and out of the room constantly. The busyness and chatter make me feel confused and detached from just about everyone and everything, except Jack and Conrad. I've turned over the note taking to Carol who is willing to help me any way she can. I just need a rest.

I retreat further. Jack seems to handle my family with the same acceptance he has always had, and though he's slow to respond and seems as confused as I feel, he's keeping up. Before this happened to

Jack I never realized how exhausting illness can be. I look at Conrad and wonder what he's feeling. I grab a post-it note and write, "This is very hard for him and me – how about you?"

"I want drugs!"

After a while I realize I have to snap out of it. As soon as I re-engage, more questions blast my brain but Trey is gone, so I write them down to ask later. Who will we call to find out what decisions were made at the Carcinoma Board? Do we have to wait for the x-ray results before Jack can put weight on his hip, or can pain be the determining factor? How do we schedule follow-up appointments with the orthopedic surgeons after Jack is discharged?

Seeing me, Carol asks, "Do you want the legal pad back?"

"No. Please. I just thought of something I need to write but I really appreciate your help. I'd like to take a few hours off from the note taking. Thanks for helping me with it." I know from the last time Jack went through the discharge process that there will be more directions than I can handle. It's a good feeling to know Carol will be another set of ears and can help me sort out what I can't keep track of and listen for information I might need and not even realize I should ask for.

I'm right. After Mary, Jack's OT, lets us know that case management will supply a shower chair, a wheelchair with left leg elevator, and a platform walker for Jack's right arm strength, Carol has the presence of mind to ask about crutches, face masks, and phone numbers to call when we're discharged.

During Jack's PT this morning he's working on transfers from the wheelchair. I have to hold his hand and elbow to help him move. Hugo reminds Jack to constantly tell his brain what he's doing as he's moving so that his brain recognizes what it's supposed to do. Jack is making progress and it's good to know that all his OT and PT will continue as an outpatient at the Medical Plaza Clinic.

CHAPTER 8

I Need Jack

I thrive on my independence. Jack and I have shared our lives wholly but we've also recognized that we have individual needs we must honor on our own. My need is traveling.

Throughout our marriage, I've traveled more without Jack than with him. He hated airports even before 9/11 when security checks made him feel like "herded cattle." I've been to New York for numerous family visits over the years. I started traveling to professional conferences all over the U.S. as soon as I became a teacher in 1992, and I've been to China twice, Costa Rica, and Canada without Jack. Our times of separation have defined our marriage as much as the times we've spent together.

I've always been confident in my ability to manage alone. Even when I found myself pregnant in January 1978, I told Jack I wouldn't marry him just because I was pregnant. Feeling like I could control my life and my decisions of how to live, I decided to just move in with Jack. If it worked out that we grew in happiness, then we could get married. If not, I could figure out my next move without being tangled in a sticky web of legal maneuvers.

My parents interfered with my independence in this particular decision. When I sent a letter to let them know I was pregnant and had decided to move to Gainesville and live with Jack, they issued an ultimatum. The words seem burned in my memory. "You have options. You can have this baby and raise it on your own. We will help you. Or you can have this baby and give it up for adoption. Or you can marry Jack and raise this baby with both its parents. But if you decide to live with Jack and not marry him, we do not want to be part of your life."

I was caught. Though I didn't want to marry Jack because I was pregnant, I was not ready to leave him either. And I certainly didn't want to do something that would divorce me from my parents.

At the time I lived in an apartment in Hyde Park, Tampa, and I worked in one of the public schools in a program for severely emotionally disturbed and autistic children. Jack was still a student at UF. It seems unbelievable in this time of ultra-communication, but back then I didn't even have a phone in my apartment. After reading the letter from my parents, I walked to the corner restaurant to use the pay phone, called Jack, and asked him to come to Tampa as soon as his classes were over the next day. When he arrived, I handed him the letter from my parents.

He was lying on my waterbed as he read. He finished the letter, wedged his arm behind his head, looked up at me and asked, "What do you want to do, Nancy?"

"I don't know, Jack, but if I have to choose between you and my parents, I will choose my parents." A month later, as we sat in Clancy's Bar in St. Pete celebrating St. Patrick's Day, Jack and I made another decision.

We got married on May 13, 1978.

As I sit in this chair wedged in the corner of Jack's hospital room, I know that if I had to make a choice between my parents and Jack again, I would choose Jack. Our marriage has had its ups and downs. There were times so difficult that I didn't think we would make it. But there were more times when my body tingled and my blood raced through my veins as Jack wrapped his strong arms around me. I always believed our marriage could make it if these highs kept getting higher while the lows dipped less.

That has happened.

Jack is my true partner in everything I do. We share decisions, listen to each other's needs, and give our best to each other. We have real conversations every single day we are together. We care about how our work and play may or may not affect the other person. We are best friends.

I've often wondered if there's some "ideal" model of what a marriage is supposed to be. For us, in order to create a self-sustaining unit, we have had to be strong together against the world, but not closed. We have had to be inclusive but not exclusive, both as individuals and as a couple. Jack and I have been alone, together, happy and sad in each other's arms. We have lifted each other out of darkness, and put each other under the spotlight of admiration.

Yes, I am strong, but how strong could I be without Jack? As our relationship has matured, our level of comfort with each other has also matured. I have learned that needing someone else does not necessarily make me weak. I need Jack. My independence was a mask. I'm dependent on Jack.

And I'm scared.

CHAPTER 9

A Primitive Cancer

Thursday, January 12, Late Morning

At 9:45 Dr. Engle makes his rounds. The results from Jack's lung biopsy confirm what was suspected – the primary cancer is lung, which has spread to other sites. If the cancer had been confined to Jack's chest, surgery would have been possible. It is not. Surgery is not an option. He confirms that gene mutation testing is being done on Jack's cells, but he doesn't hold out much hope. "The mutations are far less likely in smokers."

My heart sinks. Jack's history as a smoker becomes more of a monster every day.

Dr. Engle's comments about the radiation oncologist are more promising. "They are an excellent team. Although there is controversy about whether or not to use whole brain radiation, we at Shands prefer to target the radiation and monitor the results." The radiation that will treat Jack's hip is "Usually pretty good, and from the full bone scan, we see only one spot."

"What else?" Jack asks. The question surprises me. Clearly these brain tumors don't always interfere with Jack's thinking – he's more on target than I am.

"There may be microscopic disease elsewhere. And because this is a microscopic disease, it is hard to assess. We will use radiation on your lung for two to three weeks. We like to administer the chemo at the same time. It makes the radiation stronger. The results of the chemo aren't as good as we would like them to be, but hopefully, it will slow the progression of the disease. There is some controversy about chemo and brain radiation because of the toxicity of the drugs. So we start the chemo after the brain radiation."

Dr. Engle goes on to explain that the chemo is a two drug combination, given all in one day, and Jack will get two courses of the drug three weeks apart. They will then do a scan to see if there's shrinkage, and if so, they'll continue the chemo for four to six weeks. If the cancer is growing instead of shrinking, they'll change to an alternate drug.

Jack's cancer is a non-small cell lung cancer. It's a primitive cancer – one that is neither adenocarcinoma nor squamous cell. "It is better that it has spread to only a few sites. I'm cautiously optimistic. I would like to go after the radiation to sterilize all the met sites. After every two chemo cycles, we will reassess. We will also monitor the side effects to draw a balance between the treatment and the effects."

"Chemo cannot cure your cancer, Mr. Shelton. We have a fifty percent chance of shrinkage. Then we monitor month by month."

"What is the end game here doctor?" Jack tries again.

This time it works, and he gets an honest answer. "Patients can live one to two years with brain mets. You need to look into the Hospice program. We will allow for the most aggressive treatment. Should we decide some treatment is what you need and Hospice doesn't allow it, we will simply dis-enroll you and then re-enroll you after the treatment. I put all my patients in Hospice. It is a very positive resource. Please call *Haven Hospice* as soon as you can."

Dr. Engle pauses briefly, but then continues to explain what Jack can expect. "We will start your chemo today and your first dose will be complete before you are discharged. You will get Taxol and

Carboplatin. As an inpatient your premedication lasts five to six hours but as an outpatient it is only three to four."

"Can I go back to work?" Jack asks.

"Yes. Your hip and speech will improve. You will be able to stand and walk. The chemo will not impede you from working."

"My wife and I would like to stay here at Shands while I'm getting the radiation treatment. But what about the chemotherapy? Should we stay here in Florida until my chemo is complete?"

"I agree. You should not interrupt the radiation therapy. But the chemo is a recipe and can be done in Baltimore as well as it can be done here. Your side effects are possible fever, baldness, shortness of breath, changes in blood pressure, and you may become moody."

"For now I'm on leave from work on a week-by-week basis. But I want to get back to work when I'm able."

"You should spend as much time as you can in a chair. That will help your recovery. I will see you again before your next treatment. After you are discharged from the hospital I can see you at any time if the need arises. Your next treatment is cycle two. I want to see you in my office two days before."

"Thank you. Let's hope this works."

"Mr. Shelton, this is a difficult treatment. You have a tough tumor."

After that, what else is there to say? Hospice. Tough tumor. No cure.

But there is more to say. Stay focused. Stay positive. Thank God that Conrad, John and Carol are here.

We all decide it's a good day to go out for lunch. John and Carol have scoped out the third floor cafeteria and since Jack is learning how to transport in and out of the wheelchair, it's a perfect day for an outing. Later today Jack will get his first chemo dose and who knows how much he'll enjoy eating after that.

"Scoot forward. Toes under knees. Lean forward, nose over toes. Stand. Pivot." Yes… Jack is in the wheelchair and we're heading to the elevators.

I want to be out on the patio and John, Jack and I are looking around for a table while Carol and Conrad order our lunches. I turn towards another section of the patio and see Dr. Hyland. He's sitting at a table with extra seats. He gestures us over.

"Pull up a chair," he smiles at Jack.

"I brought my own." Jack jokes back.

"Are you sure you want my whole family at this table with you?" I ask.

"Absolutely."

Carol and Conrad show up with our food. We sit at the table talking and joking as if we were at a beachside picnic area. Dr. Hyland tells us about his wife and children, John tells Hyland about his wife and children, and Carol shares stories about her family – especially about Will and his work as a paramedic. Generally, we just have a great lunch. It's so good to feel the sun on my face, to hear Conrad laugh and to watch Jack interact with everyone. I really don't want to talk, I just want to watch and listen. When Dr. Hyland walks away from our table I'm once again reassured that staying at Shands is what we need to do. At least for now.

Once back, settled in the room, it's time to start Jack's chemo. The chemicals will run into Jack's body for hours so Jack gets comfortable on his bed and we all settle in for a few hours of socializing.

The neurology team makes a grand entrance. One of them is Dr. Cao. In the middle of this horde is Dr. Balch. We haven't met him previously but we have heard comments about the god-like attitude neurologists sometimes have. I'd say on first glance this one fits that description better than any other we've met. His gestures, posture and attitude seem to scream, "Look at me, I'm the best." He seems like the kind of man who lines the walls of his office with pictures of himself.

"How are you able to discharge Jack if his Dilantin level isn't acceptable?" I ask. This man is arrogant. I can feel his attitude and it's unsettling me.

"Mr. Shelton," Dr. Balch raises his head toward Jack, ignoring me. "We have you on 300-400 mg of Dilantin once daily. The levels we have been checking provide a guideline for how your body metabolizes the drug."

"Yes, we understand that," I respond. "But what I'm asking is how do you know that's the right dose for Jack since his levels have not stabilized? On January 10 at 1 PM his level was 0.3. He seized twice that day. At 6:30 the next day, January 11, his level was only up to 1.4, and this morning the level was only 1.1 so it is dropping again. If you discharge Jack how will we keep monitoring his level and make sure it doesn't get too low?"

"The proof is in the pudding. If he doesn't have another seizure, his levels are good."

How cold and cruel. I can't believe this man just said that. *The proof is in the pudding?* I'm stunned. Even Carol has no comeback for him. John and Jack are also silent. This man is smiling as if he's trying to be entertaining to his underlings. His efforts are spent on impressing the interns and residents crowded around him with some light, off-handed expression as a response to a very serious concern.

After the neurologists leave, Patsy, Jack's case manager, arrives with directions for discharge. She confirms the commode, the walker with attachment and wheelchair have been ordered and will be delivered. She reminds me of the dates for Jack's second chemo, before giving me a host of other information. Carol writes as I listen:

1. Take Jack's temperature twice daily. If 100.5 or above, call the number provided immediately.

2. Expect increased bruising because of the damage to Jack's platelets. Keep an eye on this side effect and show Dr. Engle if bruising is excessive.

3. Use break through pain meds for any aches and pains. It's very important to "stay ahead of the pain."

4. Side effects take three to four days to appear and include aches and pains, tingling in hands and feet, loose stools, and ringing in ears.

5. Days ten through fourteen (after the chemo) are the highest risk days for temperature elevation.

6. There's a small chance of delayed nausea.

7. Eat anything you want – all of it. High calorie foods like ice cream and milk shakes are good.

8. The platins in the drugs may change your taste but just keep trying different foods – it's very important to keep your weight up.

All these people come and go while Jack is hooked up to the machine that continues to pump poison into his bloodstream. A new normal has crept into our lives and taken possession of our minds and our habits. I look out the window and turn my thoughts to Payne's Prairie that spreads out from my window and goes on for miles in its flat green vastness. It's a geological landmark but to me it's a wonder. When I was a kid living in the mountainous region of Upstate New York, like all school children I had to learn about various land formations. It was virtually impossible for me to conceptualize a prairie and the peaceful feeling of looking out over one. When I first moved to Gainesville I marveled at the buffalo roaming the prairie. The small herd was sometimes visible from Highway 441, and when Conrad was young I would pull over so we could watch the majestic animals graze. In 1986 when Halley's Comet's perihelion granted us a sky-show, Conrad, Aaron, Chad, Becky and I came to the prairie to watch.

Over the centuries, the prairie has flooded and naturally drained which has allowed it to become a lake and then return to itself – a prairie. I turn from the window and pray to the gods of science and nature, "Please return my dear Jack to himself too."

Friday, January 13

It's Friday the 13th. A day to celebrate. Our family number is 13 and Jack and I love Friday the 13th. For us it's always a good day, especially when May 13 falls on a Friday. It happens a lot and I always joke that it's not a coincidence that our wedding anniversary is on a day other people think is for crazies.

Up until now, we have felt lucky. Jack has not experienced side effects from the chemo. With his appetite still strong, he welcomes the breakfast served this morning, reaching first for the orange juice. This reprieve was not meant to last. As soon as the juice flows down, it rushes back up again flooding away any hope for a lucky streak on this Friday the 13th. I spend the next hour by his side, holding the hospital-pink vomit catcher and a series of washcloths to wipe his face, which is turning more pallid with every retching convulsion. John and Carol are here and I can see how difficult it is for them to find the right words – to try to feel comfortable in a discomforting situation. They can only stay for a brief visit because Carol is going to Tampa to pick up her eldest daughter, Nancy Lee, and John is driving back to New York.

The rest of the morning is focused on discharge. This includes Jack learning how to get in and out of the car. In preparation for the lessons, Conrad drives the car from our home to the hospital. Kiley has followed in her vehicle and, leaving us with the car keys, Kiley and Conrad take our belongings home.

I try to be excited but a heaviness bears down on my mind, not letting me feel good about this discharge. It's sort of like when I'm driving and the traffic light is on yellow – I know it will quickly turn red and then I'll instantaneously have to decide whether to step on the gas or slam on the brakes. But today's problem is that I'm not the one who's driving. If I were, I'd be slamming on the brakes. Instead, whoever *is* driving is stepping on the gas.

Once again, we experience a revolving door of white coats, one after another repeating the same information. Once again, the summative paragraph on Jack's discharge instructions packs a week of trauma into too few words:

> *Mr. Shelton you were admitted due to recurrent hip pain. We first treated you with pain medications and evaluated your hip with Imaging. It was found on imaging that there was indeed a metastatic lesion from the Lung cancer that was diagnosed previously. Radiology oncology was consulted and they went ahead with Radiation therapy to the hip. During the course of your stay after scheduled radiotactic surgery you had recurrent seizures. You were on anti seizure medicines but your body metabolizes it much quicker and the dose needed to be increased, which you will continue. Physical therapy recommended continued care when you are home which we provided for you and they will call you when they will be going to your home. Dr. Engle decided as well to get started on Chemotherapy with Taxol. You had mild nausea and vomiting the next morning which is a side effect of the treatment. I will provide you anti-nausea medication to take home. You will continue radiation therapy to the hip and chemo treatment when followed by Dr. Engle. We have set an Orthopedic appointment for you to have follow up on your leg. In the mean time we provided you pain medications and Physical therapy.*

I've never wanted to be a nurse. I hate anything related to the human body. I didn't even teach human biology to my elementary students when I was a classroom teacher – I made my interns do it. That's all coming back to haunt me because I feel totally incompetent to take care of Jack once we're discharged.

The hiccups have been steadily ravishing Jack's body for hours on end for the past few weeks and scare the hell out of me. But, beyond that, I'm petrified at missing a piece of the convoluted mess of instructions we have been given and making a terrible, irrevocable mistake. What if I screw up his meds? What if I miss taking his temperature, and he gets really sick before we even know he has a fever and it gets too late to fight the infection? Though I would never admit it to Jack, I am also terrified at what his body will throw at us next. I'm afraid he'll vomit more from the chemo and I won't be able to get him to eat. I'm afraid he'll get constipated. More than anything, I'm afraid Jack will have another seizure.

At 11:42 AM Jack is discharged.

We're set free. But are we? How do I act? What do I say? I have to think before making every move and forming every syllable. So does Jack but for different reasons – his are physical, mine are emotional.

Armed with Jack's wheelchair, several lessons on how to "transfer" in and out of the car, a fistful of prescriptions, a collection of random medical supplies, an exhaustive chemo schedule, radiation and follow-up medical appointments, and the last of our personal belongings, we are loaded up and I steer my little Benz away from the Davis Cancer Center.

I'm afraid to drive. Just a few weeks ago this car was the focus of my thoughts. My Christmas present from Jack. It brought rich excitement to our holiday. Today, it's just a car. One I am not sufficiently familiar with to feel confident that I "know" well enough to avoid doing anything that might jar Jack's hip. With a death grip on the steering wheel, I search for bumps in the road, stay two car lengths away from the nearest vehicle, drive under the speed limit and try to act normal. The problem is, I don't remember what normal is.

I don't know what Jack is thinking and though I want to know, I don't dare ask. Desperately racking my brain for a safe way to proceed, I wonder if I can use Jack's affinity for the comfort of familiar routines to help ease the tension I'm feeling. I force myself to recall previous trips home from various hospital stays and offer what I remember.

"Do you want to go directly home or would you like to be out for a while?" I ask.

"I want to go home."

"Okay. Should we stop at the pharmacy on our way and fill your scripts or would you rather I take you home and then go back out after them?"

"Let's stop on the way. We can use the drive-through so I don't have to get out of the car, right?"

It should be easy, but when we get to CVS, we are instantly submerged into the dark abyss that sometimes comes with independence. The pharmacist servicing the drive-up window won't fill Jack's prescription for his morphine. The realization that we are being rejected sinks in, driving an unexpected sharp nail in my already pummeled psyche. I'm short and the car sits low, much lower than the drive-thru service window. My diminutive physical position is not helping my argument. I step out of the car, stand at the window and ask to speak to the head pharmacist.

When the head pharmacist appears at the window a couple of minutes later, I make my case. "My husband has just been discharged from Shands. He has stage four cancer and he's in pain." As his expression travels the surprisingly short road from annoyance to compassion, I gulp and continue, "The doctor wrote out the month and said that it meets the law requiring words and not numerals. I need this prescription filled," I push out, focusing on the words to control the break in my voice lurking at the back of my throat. "I need it filled before my husband's pain increases. Please call the hospital," I plead, "they will confirm this and fax what you need. I'm sure they will help you." I look into the pharmacist eyes, willing for concession to appear. "We just drove directly from Shands – here's the number for the floor. Ask to speak to Dr. Ruiz or Dr. Hyland."

But, though the compassion stayed put, the concession I was hoping for never made it to the pharmacist's eyes. "I'm sorry Mrs. Shelton. We can't use a fax. We must have an original," he says kindly but firmly with the air of a professional citing a firm rule. "I'm sorry your husband's doctor doesn't know the regulation but it's new this January 1 and I can't make an exception. Morphine is a heavily controlled narcotic. I must have the prescription written correctly and it must be an original."

As I have done so many times since Terrible Tuesday, I call Conrad and pass this problem on to him to solve. I know from my work in education that when people are emotionally upset, their cognitive abilities diminish. I'm not mad at myself, at Jack, at the doctor, at the pharmacy or even at the law. But I'm mad. Jack needs his meds.

An hour later Kiley drives into our driveway, walks into the house, hands me Jack's meds and smiles. She left work when Conrad called her, drove to 8 East, picked up the correctly written prescription, and had it filled at CVS.

As if just having cancer isn't challenging enough, being home means we must find a way to function with some semblance of normalcy. I don't want to live at Shands but I also don't want Jack to feel like he's a burden. I don't know what he's thinking and we've been married long enough for me to know he'll tell me if and when he's ready.

Conrad grills a steak for dinner, and afterwards, as we are cleaning up, Jack navigates himself to the kitchen to where the coffee maker is set up.

"Hump." Always a man of few words, he sits pondering the location of all the things he needs to set up the coffee. Conrad, who often reads Jack's mind more accurately than I, is watching him.

"Dad, I think I need to move that for you."

"Would you son?"

"Sure. Just give me a minute. I have a plan."

Conrad sets up a side table in a place where Jack can reach it. Then Conrad sets the coffee machine on the table with the coffee, filters, and a few mugs. Jack's way to show his love is to cook for us, to set up coffee on an alarm so that every morning we are treated with his service to us, and to quietly just go about taking care of what needs to be done. It takes Jack almost forty-five minutes to set up the coffee with one arm, sitting in a wheelchair, but he does it.

We watch *Harry Potter and the Deathly Hallows, Part I*, and then Conrad helps me transfer Jack from the wheelchair to the bed. When I finally get into bed, I'm more emotionally exhausted than physically spent, but I still can't sleep worth a damn. I wake up every single time Jack moves and every time I have to move. Jack's body is weak. I can't trust it. I can't move with ease because I don't want to bump him and hurt him.

CHAPTER 10

Home And Back, Again

Saturday, January 14

It's Saturday, but there's no time to slow down. At 9:00 AM Jack's home therapist arrives. Jack is determined he'll get his hand working and his coordination back and doesn't want to go a single day without therapy. I sit with the therapist, Matt, through all the insurance and scheduling discussions. When Matt is ready to start Jack's therapy, he asks, "Who will be helping you carry through with your exercises on the off days that I'm not here? Will it be your wife or your son?"

It takes a long time for Jack to find his words, but in this case, he uses his eyes as his first response. He looks directly to Conrad who is already in motion, walking from the kitchen to Jack and Matt, who are in the dining room. I have no idea if Jack and Conrad discussed this earlier, but I have clearly been replaced. I'm so relieved. I need to pass some responsibility to Conrad and he's more than willing to accept it.

Not so long ago, before I began to understand how cancer ruins a life, I took it for granted that Jack and I would always be able to enjoy an active lifestyle. I've always suspected that Jack's internal organs could not be as healthy as mine. One of his favorite quotes, which he says with a sheepish grin illuminating his face, is "Live fast, die young and leave a good-looking corpse." In our younger days we both consumed our share of alcohol, Jack smoked more than his share of pot, and Jack's steaks have often been said to be more like a side of beef than a dinner-sized meal. But I never anticipated he'd be stricken down so fast and so young. I was the one with so many ailments. So much so that Jack named me "Hurts Rankie" when we started dating.

Every single thing Jack does takes so much energy, and he has a very limited supply. This morning he's exhausted after his PT session and Conrad helps him transfer into his bed for a nap. I climb up onto the bed and sit with Jack until I hear his breathing change and I'm sure he's asleep. Quietly I shift off the bed, tiptoe out of the room, and pull the door almost closed as I head to the kitchen.

"What else needs to be done?" I ask Kiley as she prepares the cheese tray.

"Check the list. I don't know how long it's going to take your parents to get here. We can never tell what the traffic coming up *I-75* will be."

"Well, you're right about that," I say as I start making the iced tea. "But either Carol or Nancy Lee will be driving so the trip will be a little shorter than if my parents were trying to drive it alone. Not that they could – I think by the time you're in your eighties you deserve to be chauffeured."

"Sad to say, but it's great that it's your father's birthday next week and Carol and her daughter planned a visit. Your parents can come to see Jack without the burden of driving." Kiley is right. My parents wouldn't be able to make the trip without Carol and Nancy Lee.

We're ordering a barbeque lunch but there's still a lot of work to be done. I leave the kitchen to put the plates, silverware and napkins out, wash the tables and then take the dogs out in the back yard for a walk. I want them tired when everyone arrives.

I feel peaceful in this yard where I am surrounded by green and feel the vast openness of nature. Jack and I have the field adjacent to our yard mowed once a month so it doesn't become overgrown. The centuries-old live oak tree with swaying Spanish moss stands quiet and steady, spreading from the sky to the ground as a symbol of almighty power. In the distance a tee box for the golf course reminds me of a more care-free time when Conrad golfed regularly and teased his father and me because we have a house on a golf course when neither of us golf.

Kiley has finished setting out several hors d'oeuvres and heads out to the porch to arrange the chairs. Conrad has finished vacuuming and sweeping and shifts his attention to the laundry room. I focus on the bathroom – shining the sink and scrubbing the toilet.

Jack wakes up from his nap. Conrad stops shuffling the laundry from the washer to the dryer to help Jack get ready for our company.

Jack's right arm is so weak that he has to hold it in place or it slides off his lap and hangs off the side of the wheelchair. Conrad has fashioned a sling of sorts for him, and that, together with a pillow that Jack snuggles onto his lap, helps. But as much as he tries, his arm still slides to the side. Jack looks uncomfortable. He looks weak. And sick. I wonder how much it affects Conrad to see his father suffering with this disease.

Everyone is here and there's a lot of action. Our Florida home is relatively new, and neither Carol nor Nancy Lee has been here before so we spend time and positive energy showing it off. Nancy Lee is lively. She's Skyped in her husband, Sean, and daughter Hannah, and is giving them a tour of our house too. God – this new generation with their digital communication is draining for me. What happened to a good old-fashioned visit with tea and cookies? I hate having my voice recorded and I'm not all that thrilled to have my picture taken and blasted all over the universe.

Nancy Lee is a Tebow fan and she's brought Jack a Denver Tebow shirt. She also brought two Gator rival shirts to tease him with – the Georgia Bull Dawgs and the Texas Longhorns. I swear more pictures are taken of Jack in these few hours than have ever been snapped in any other two-hour span during his whole life. It makes me feel nervous – like Jack is on display. I know that's not anyone's intent but I can't relax at all. I make a note:

Anxiety

Anxiety's skin is stretched tightly across her face. She is sweating. Her heart is racing. Confidence drains from her heart and drips off her trembling hands. Trying not to be exposed, *Anxiety* moves to the corner of the room hoping to go unnoticed by those around her. But her painful uneasiness wafts through the air around her. *Fear* smells it and closes in but, if *Anxiety* is lucky, *Compassion* cuts in first offering a quiet walk and a gentle touch on the shoulder.

Carol and I make eye contact. Speaking no words we communicate with each other – we need time alone. I quietly rise from the couch and walk through the living room, out the French doors, and onto the porch. Carol hesitates just a minute so that no one realizes we're leaving the house together. As soon as Carol starts moving from the kitchen towards the dining room, I walk to the screen door on the porch. I move with purpose, head down, quick pace, until I'm in the middle of my back yard.

"Well, we pulled that one off," Carol chuckles as she reaches me in the yard.

"Yea. I can't take much more talking," I respond.

Never one to dwell on conversation about feelings, Carol let's my comment go and skillfully talks at length about how peaceful my yard is, how quiet the neighborhood, and how much land the dogs have to run. She doesn't barrage me with questions or make comments about Jack. She just tries to make the afternoon a little bit less tense.

It's a relatively short visit in normal terms, but a long time for Jack to be attentive and interacting. When Carol, Nancy Lee and my parents head back to Hillsborough County it's already 4:00 PM. Once again, Jack is exhausted. Conrad helps him to our room and back into bed.

Wanting to be close to Jack, I slide between the sheets on my side of the bed and pick up my book. I'm not usually a series reader, but I mentally thank Vince Flynn for the many volumes in the Mitch Rapp storyline, and my brother John for introducing them to me a few months ago.

After about an hour I set my book aside and lie down to feel close to Jack. He seems to be in a deep sleep. I watch him, my hand resting on his chest and our bodies touching in our natural way. I set my mind to work recalling as many images of us as I can – Jack and me on his boat on Lake Santé Fe, Jack hanging off the top of the Maya ruins in Belize in a pose that would convince any viewer that he's falling, Jack bundled up in his snowsuit shoveling snow, laughing and playing with Meghan and Ben during the 2010 blizzard, Jack and I with Pat and Sue fishing in the Gulf, Jack manning the grill at Conrad's high school baseball field, Jack standing out on the rock ledge at Augur Falls with Carol and Bill last Easter.

I drift off to sleep, my mind filled with pleasant memories.

SHIT! I bolt up in the bed. JACK IS SEIZING AGAIN! I yell out for Kiley and Conrad. They rush into the room.

"Kiley please time the seizure." I know the doctors will ask us the duration of the episode.

Conrad and I try to hold Jack steady. This seizure is the first Kiley and Conrad see. It's the worst since the first.

Finally, Jack's body stops twitching, his eyes stop darting back and forth, his leg stops jerking and his arm relaxes.

When Jack tries to speak, he cannot. He tries to move his right arm but he cannot. "Can you move your leg?" He's still.

After what seems like an eternity but I am sure is only minutes, Jack is able to make sounds that should be speech, but they are not. He sounds totally wrong. His pitch is off worse than before. His syllables are abrupt and truncated. He can't push two words against each other – there are spaces and pauses between every word and sometimes between syllables.

"My head hurts," he manages to utter.

"I need to call the doctor."

With long pauses between words, Jack says, "I'm afraid of what these seizures are doing to me." The effort it takes for Jack to say this makes me even more afraid.

"Jack, we need help." I don't move. I don't know what to do.

"My head hurts."

"Jack, let me just send a note to Alexander and see what we should do, okay?"

Conrad doesn't wait for an answer. "What's his email address, Mom? I'll send it."

I stay beside Jack. Time passes. Jack doesn't feel better and, unlike previous seizures, he hasn't regained movement with the passage of time.

"Mom, I think you should call and not wait for an email."

I manage to get a call through to Dr. Narain. The answer is not what I had hoped. The additional damage and the pain Jack is feeling in his head isn't good. We need to get back to the ER. I ask Dr. Narain if there's any way we can be admitted without having to go through the ER.

"The best is to call the ambulance. The ER works more effectively for people who come in the ambulance than those who are driven in private cars."

"I have little hope. Jack's previous ER runs were via ambulance and last week Jack spent twelve hours in excruciating pain before they gave him any drugs." What I don't say to Dr. Narain is that even if Jack can manage one more trip to the ER, I am not sure I can. I'm emotionally depleted. Physically inert. Mentally empty.

"I'm so sorry Mrs. Shelton. I know this is difficult. Please call the floor when you get to the ER and we'll do what we can to help you."

The EMTs on Rescue 9 are the same team who brought Jack to the hospital last week. They clearly care about him, their voices and movements are gentle as they move Jack from the vehicle to the ER. As soon as Jack is situated, I call up to 8 East. There *are* angels in our world because just after I make the call, someone comes down from 8 East and rather than wait for all the "necessary procedures," she pushes Jack's wheelchair away from the waiting area towards the elevators.

We are back on 8 East.

Sunday, January 15

Jack's condition is worse. Being back at the hospital feels even more defeating than our previous re-admission. It's Sunday so there are few people here. Besides that, it's mid-month so the Attending Physician will change and Jack will no longer have Dr. Hyland as his over-all caregiver. We will have to start a relationship with yet another oncologist.

We're in a different room this time, but it's in the same general location and we still have a beautiful view of Payne's Prairie. Gratefully, we still have the same group of nurses.

Jack's hiccups are relentless. None of the meds we have tried have been able to make them stop. Jack's chest hurts. He feels beaten. He can't make them stop. He can't complete a sentence without expulsions of air and muscle spasms interrupting him. He's completely unable to relax. And because of his pain and defeat, I feel tense and desperate every time I hear the distinct sound a hiccup makes as it is emitted from his body.

Jack's relationship with Pat and Sue is more like family than it is a friendship. Jack's father and Pat's father worked together when the kids were young – one owned a contracting business, the other a paving company. Sue and Jack have been friends since middle school. Pat and Sue were high school sweethearts.

After Jack moved to Gainesville, before and after our marriage, Pat and Sue's house was Jack's "home" base. We spent holidays together, went fishing, water skiing, and diving every chance we could get. Our kids grew up more like cousins than friends and that's still true. Jack is their daughter Kelly's godfather.

Eventually Pat and Sue moved off the beach to Crystal River. We were geographically much closer and our visits increased in frequency. Sue and I became friends, independent of our husbands.

No matter what life threw our way, nothing came between Jack's friendship with Pat and Sue. When their son Adam tragically died at age 15, we wouldn't leave them alone and insisted visits were necessary. After 33 years of marriage, when Pat and Sue got divorced, Jack and I stayed friends with them both, consciously sharing time with each of them as they set out on individual paths in life. When Jack and I moved to Maryland, we made visits to Crystal River every time we came south – never missing a chance to go fishing, to swim with the manatees, or just to share a meal with our friends.

Since Jack's seizure he has spoken to Pat and Sue three or four times and I've sent an email or two, but we haven't really been able to communicate too much.

When Pat walks into Jack's room Conrad just bursts out laughing. True to form, Pat is making a fashion statement. It's his signature – sometimes it's a pair of shorts that clash wildly with his shirt, an article of clothing from another century, or a wild wig. Today it's his snakeskin belt and matching cowboy boots. The funny thing is that no matter how peculiar Pat dresses, he still seems to look nice.

Pat walks directly to Jack and gives him a hug. Kelly follows. I'm so glad Conrad is with us because he's able to make the conversation stay alive. It's difficult for me to watch Jack reassure Pat that he's "coming back – just wait and see." Kelly and Conrad take a walk, I'm sure so Kelly won't cry in front of Jack.

Jack's speech has deteriorated. He can't finish a sentence. His voice sounds like he's mentally challenged. He doesn't want to speak and keeps apologizing because of how he sounds. He can't find his words but he does his best to interact.

Visits drain Jack's energy. After Pat and Kelly leave, Jack naps. I turn to my book to see what Mitch Rapp is up to.

At 3:10 PM Jack's door opens. I see the neurologist, Dr. Cao. I quickly set my book aside and walk towards him to stop him from approaching Jack. He's with Alexander, which calms me a bit, but I know he's a neurologist and I'm still raging inside because of Dr. Balch's aloofness and the consequences Jack has paid for not having more critical care concerning his Dilantin levels. Two other people in white coats I don't know are behind Alexander.

"I do not want Dr. Balch near my husband."

"Dr. Shelton, what's wrong?" Alexander asks.

"I specifically asked Dr. Balch how he was going to make sure Jack's Dilantin levels were sufficient and he, in a very cocky tone, said, '*The proof is in the pudding.*' That is not the kind of medical approach we want and I don't want him, his partners, or anyone associated with him to treat my husband." I let my words hang in the air, supported by the glare I direct at Dr. Cao.

Dr. Cao respects my stance, allowing the silence to punctuate my anger before he responds. "I can assure you that is not the approach I will use. I cannot speak for Dr. Balch, but I will do my very best to get Mr. Shelton's seizures under control."

I step aside and let him go to Jack. The weakness in Jack's arm, leg and hand are significantly worse, and he can't even move his right leg. He can't spell backwards nor can he do a simple math subtraction problem that involves making change from a dollar. These are all tasks he was able to do every other time he was tested, and there have been many such occasions when Jack's cognitive abilities have been tested since Terrible Tuesday.

Dr. Cao says something about right lateral damage and that he will check the MRI. He increases Jack's Dilantin to 150 mg three times a day and adds Keppra twice a day to his regimen. Jack has been loaded with Keppra via the IV. Dr. Cao explains that Dilantin has a 32-hour half-life and it takes four to five days to get a patient in a therapeutic range.

After the physicians leave, Jack falls asleep. For an hour he doesn't hiccup.

As soon as Jack wakes up, the hiccups return.

Bill and Danling come by with more food for us tonight. They have brought another container of dumplings and two other dishes Danling knows Jack likes. Jack has already had his dinner but it wouldn't have mattered, he appreciates the food but he won't eat in front of Danling and Bill. He needs too much help. He's made progress using his left hand, but in order to improve his coordination and repair the damage caused by the seizures, he needs to use his right. He has special flatware with thick handles that the OT has provided. He can grip those better but it's a laborious process.

I have no trouble using my chopsticks and eating while the dinner is hot. I know Jack wants me to. He's not able to converse much at all. Bill and Danling stay for only a short visit.

Monday, January 16

This morning we meet the new attending oncologist, Dr. Binh Tran. He's ordering another MRI to check for swelling and breakthrough bleeding. He's continuing orders to monitor Jack's Dilantin levels. Dr. Tran has no magic cure for Jack's hiccups, which, as usual, are a constant irritant, but he suggests a new drug we have not yet tried, Reglan. Jack has started taking it and we're not trying any other drug for 48 hours in hopes that the Reglan will work – if not immediately, then over time.

I'm devastated when I see that Jack is developing a bedsore. Bedsores to me mean a patient has been neglected. My association with bedsores is related to elderly, semiconscious nursing home patients who are left to die in desolate, lonely facilities. My husband, who

I have tried so hard to take care of, should NOT have a bedsore.

Carla, Jack's nurse, says I have done everything possible for Jack and that I should not feel responsible. But I do.

Grief is exhausting. It's terrifying. Hiding my grief is the only way I can steady myself against the torrent of pain that flushes through my body when I let myself acknowledge Jack is dying in front of my eyes.

I bare my soul only to a few people. Fear keeps me from revealing myself. I don't allow myself the luxury of truth because once words are spoken they cannot be silenced.

I'll do anything necessary so that I don't lose control of the tone of the interactions between me and my parents and my siblings. If I show them my pain I will lose that control. The Sheltons and the Rankies are the most important people in my life. To stay strong in front of them I cannot reveal my innermost fear. So I expose it to only a few people.

When Danling and I are together, words aren't necessary. Silently, I let her see into my soul. I write emails to Pandora and tell her Jack is dying. On the phone I tell Becky I don't know how I'll live without Jack. I ask Morna to find Jack's Last Will and Testament because I realize that I'm the one who needs to "get our affairs in order." I ask Carol to make arrangements in case the "end game" stuns us.

For the first time in my life I'm grateful that Jack's mother was such a bitch to us. It's because of her that Jack and I have wills.

Jack earned his degree from UF on August 9, 1979. We were both really proud of his accomplishment. He had made the decision to be a scientist and managed to find a way to get through college. His childhood friends were boat builders, fishermen, drug smugglers and in the construction business. But Jack knew what he wanted and though it took him six years, he made it to his goal.

Jack didn't participate in the formal graduation ceremony. Instead we planned an excursion to both Tampa and St. Pete to celebrate with our friends. I had squirreled away enough money to treat Jack to dinner at Bern's Steakhouse in Tampa. Bern's is still, to this day, one of the most unique dining experiences Jack and I have shared together. The decorations are gaudy, or they were back in 1979, but the food was unbelievable. The restaurant supplied its own produce from a farm they owned, the beef was so tender it barely needed to be chewed, and the staff all worked several years on the farm or in the kitchen before becoming wait staff.

My friends in Tampa agreed to babysit for Conrad while Jack and I dined. Conrad, 11 months old by then, had been a most efficient crawler. He used to bear crawl at top speed, out-motoring some toddlers who were in a full run but he was still not walking. He had never been with a "babysitter," having only been left for short periods of time with our friends who he knew well, and I was nervous about leaving him. He didn't know Rose or Terry. To make myself feel better about leaving him, I put all of Conrad's favorite toys out on the floor and Jack and I hung around Terry's house long enough to let Conrad start playing. Finally, we had to leave – our dinner reservations couldn't wait for a young mother to ease her anxiety any longer. Just as we were ready to go, Conrad stood up in the midst of his toys and walked seven steps over to his father, hugged Jack's legs, and then plopped back down on the floor, giggling. It made our night of celebration even more significant than it already was.

Our friends shared our joy in many ways that week. But not Jack's mother. Her words were the expected ones of "congratulations" and "I'm proud of you" but her subsequent actions were shocking. She handed Jack a bill for what she determined was her cost of raising him from the time of her second marriage, when Jack was barely a teenager, until Jack and I were married in 1978. I can't even explain the shock we felt, and for Jack, the embarrassment. The bill was almost $10,000. Even Jack, who is non-confrontational, rarely disagreeing and never arguing with others, was appalled.

Jack asked his mother how she determined the amount of money she wanted reimbursed. As evidence, she provided him with a stack of cancelled checks. These checks dated back more than a decade. They covered doctor appointments, eyeglasses, books, clothes, and other normal expenses parents are encumbered with providing for their children. They also included car insurance and a few junior college tuition payments.

Sadly, Jack took the checks and went through them one by one. He found, mixed into the pile, several written to doctors he had never seen. To insurance companies he never had heard of. Jack assumed they were bills from his brother, mixed in either intentionally or accidentally. Everything Jack didn't recognized he sent back to his mother. The remainder totaled over $7,000. He agreed to pay this money back to his mother.

I was furious. Who ever heard of paying your parents for your childhood expenses? We had no money. Jack didn't even have a job yet. But Jack refused to argue with his mother, and she was demanding payment.

There was no way I was going to be responsible for these payments. So we went to the Legal Aid Society where we could get free legal services and Jack had a promissory note written that stated he, not I, would be responsible to give his mother this money. The lawyers advised us that it didn't matter what was written in the promissory note, as Jack's wife I would be held responsible if Jack signed the note.

Afraid of what Jack's mother might do next, Jack and I also decided we had better get wills written. At that time I had no family living in the State of Florida. Should Jack and I be killed in an accident, the courts would naturally have awarded custody of Conrad to Jack's family before mine – they were Florida residents. So, poor as we were with absolutely no financial assets, we both had wills written to secure custody of our son. I had it written in the wills that I would not be liable to pay Jack's mother even though the provision would not have held up in court.

I know exactly where our wills are. Morna will go to our house and read Jack's for me. I need to make sure it's as I remember – that everything just goes to me should Jack pre-decease me. In my darkest moments I know that's coming.

This afternoon we meet Dr. Howard. He recommends increasing the dose of the steroids Jack is on in order to help with the edema in Jack's brain. The MRI results indicate that the tumor is the culprit causing the seizures. "The seizures are symptoms of the irritation caused by the stereotactic surgery."

Dr. Howard explains that Jack's brain needs to "reset itself" after the seizures and it may take longer because it becomes harder after each seizure. This seizure was longer than the second and third. "I'm concerned that the small focal seizures could spread and become more involved, and eventually lead to unconsciousness." This news is just not good. The more Jack's brain swells, the longer his recovery period. The more seizures he has, the more likely he is to have more.

Everything about the seizures concerns Jack and me. While John and Carol were visiting, John outright asked Jack what the seizures felt like. Jack told him, "They feel like a giant charley horse. They start on the right side then move across my body to the other side all the while I'm wondering if it's going to get my heart and that will be the end."

Respecting Jack's knowledge as a genetic researcher, Dr. Howard explains the science behind his treatment. The class of drugs for treating seizures is 2Y2 and is NCI approved. Cytochrome P450 (CYP 450) enzymes are used to metabolize drugs, and the genetic variability in the enzymes can influence how a patient responds. It seems that CYP 450 enzymes have played a role in how Jack metabolizes the Dilantin.

Although it's difficult for him to get his question out, Jack's brain is working well enough for him to ask about a metabolic panel for Single Nucleotides Polymorphism (SNPs). Jack and Jing have run thousands of these specific gene arrays that target over 2000 SNPs (mutations) in CYP450 and other genes associated with a person's ability to metabolize drugs. His lab has done studies that lead to implementing one specific test looking at which patient populations can and cannot metabolize the anticoagulant Plavix, one of the most widely prescribed drugs. Jack knows metabolic profiling is possible. It's one of the areas of patient care that will be developed in the very near future. In fact, metabolic profiling will become a routine test for patients who enter the hospital. The growth of personalized medicine can greatly benefit patient care. This is what Jack's boss, Alan, the Associate Dean for Personalized and Genomic Medicine, is known for and what Jack's work in the lab at UMB contributes to when it comes to the advancement of health care in the United States.

Personalized medicine in practice, at least at Shands, has not caught up with scientific knowledge. Dr. Howard tells Jack that it's not common practice at this point to run a SNP for Jack, and that their treatment choice is to see how Jack responds to Keppra.

As I listen to the two men, trying to understand them, I make a decision – I'm calling Steve. Back in 2007 Jack had a lot of pain in his legs when he walked that was eventually diagnosed as a symptom related to a back injury he sustained as a teenager. Before Jack turned to a neurosurgeon, he sought advice from Steve, who is a neurologist and my research partner's husband. Tonight I'm going to ask Steve to explain as much as he can without having examined Jack or his records. Given the scientific knowledge about CYP 450, I don't understand why they didn't immediately consider a different anti-seizure drug for Jack. I don't understand why they would discharge him from the hospital without knowing his Dilantin level was safe.

I've never been a patient person in conversation with Jack. We have two completely different discourse patterns. I have no trouble with overlapping speech. Jack considers all attempts to join in a conversation "butting in." Sometimes I stop myself and try to converse his way, but mostly I have continued just being me, talking when I want, figuring it's his problem if he can't adjust. But now I will not answer for Jack, I will not finish his sentences when he's searching for his words, and I will not start speaking while he's speaking. I don't know if it's the panic in me that is surfacing as patience, but

I know I'm more patient with Jack than I have ever been.

"Jack, I want to talk to Steve. I don't really understand what's going on with your seizures and I want to ask him what his opinion is. Is that okay with you?"

As he tries in vain to speak, I find myself fighting off tears. "It's more than okay. I want to know what he thinks too." Just these two short sentences took energy for him to articulate. I sit down on the edge of Jack's bed.

Thankfully, Steve is home. He's willing to talk to us, but does caution us that he doesn't have Jack's records and can only share his thoughts that are not true medical opinions because he's not here and can't examine Jack. But that's enough for us.

"Steve, the neurologists use language they think I understand but I don't. I need more details than they give. What is a focal seizure?" As I ask this question, I feel Jack's one good hand reach up and warm my back.

"That's just a seizure when only one part of the brain is involved."

I explain Jack's inability to use his right hand. As I say this, I lean gently back against Jack. I'm careful because I don't want to bump into any part of his medical equipment, but Jack has reached out to touch me and I want to feel closer to him while I talk. As Jack feels my movement, he instinctively eases his hand around my body.

Steve answers me, and though it's through a cell phone and we are hundreds of miles away from each other, I feel Steve's concern for Jack. "He probably has left brain involvement. That affects his language and his right arm/hand."

Though I really don't want to emphasize Jack's weaknesses when Jack can hear me, I know I have to be honest with Steve if I want him to share his knowledge with us. So I ask what I would rather not have to ask in front of Jack. "Jack is confused, he's unable to understand directions to move different parts of his body. Will his brain heal?"

I'm fully resting on Jack. His hand is on my chest and I feel as close to Jack as I have ever felt. I know Jack understands everything I have said and can also hear Steve's responses.

"It's very unusual to have permanent damage. His arm will come back. His brain has been overly active and when that happens sometimes it just goes to sleep for a while. If the damage is all caused by the seizures, he should fully recover. It will take time, but it will heal."

Hearing Steve's encouraging assessment makes me realize I have done the right thing in letting Jack hear the whole conversation. So I continue. "Should they test for new lesions?"

"I can't say, but the odds are it's just a seizure caused by what we already know."

"What about permanent damage? The doctor said he's concerned that Jack's seizures will become more involved and more dangerous." As I ask these questions I can't help but to wonder why the conversations with the neurologists here at Shands are so stressful. I think Steve must have a gift beyond what other doctors have and his humanness is extraordinary.

"A seizure has to last thirty minutes or more to cause permanent damage. In an otherwise healthy brain, the patient comes back in ten to twenty minutes. But with an abnormality, as with Jack's cancer and radiation, it can take days. Do you know where Jack's lesions are?"

"I think near the cortex and the frontal parietal lobes. But I don't know what that means."

"Maybe you can contact Patient Care, Complaints and Concerns at the hospital and ask them to Fax Jack's records to me. I'll take a look at them and see if I can tell how much tissue was damaged. It has to be beyond a certain threshold for permanent damage. If they send the records I'll review them for you."

I thank Steve, and he gives the phone to Bess. We are not only research partners, but also friends. I continue to lie back on Jack's bed and Bess and I talk about other things besides Jack's cancer. I feel relaxed. My head is on Jack's belly, he's stroking my cheek and running his fingers through my hair. As I get ready to hang up, Bess says, "Tell Jack we love him."

"Love you too." Jack says. I turn my phone off, and continue lying against Jack. I feel a kind of peace that's almost tranquility – but not quite. I don't say it to Jack, but I no longer trust his body will behave. I know, deep in my heart, that he's only going to be with me for a quantifiable number of days.

I finally sit up and turn to face Jack. He's crying. In all the years we have been married I have seen Jack cry once before. He was 25 years old and feeling sorry for himself because he was married, had a child, and didn't have the freedom his friends at UF had. I didn't understand his flood of emotion that day and I am equally confused tonight. "What's wrong? Did I hurt you?" I ask, fearing I had caused Jack pain by lying on him.

Jack realizes he needs to speak. It takes him forever to articulate his thoughts but when he does, the message is a good one. "I could hear Steve on the phone. I was so relieved to hear his voice. And to know I can get my body to work again. These are tears of joy."

Amazingly, Jack has had only a few hiccupping episodes all afternoon. Before falling asleep, we take a moment to appreciate the stillness of his body.

Tuesday, January 17

Dr. Engle wants Jack discharged. He's here this morning with reassurance that Jack can be treated as an outpatient even though his "disease is *difficult*."

"The seizures are caused by the disease in your brain. Any swelling makes a difference and in your case there is a lot of swelling from the treatment. There is no room for swelling or inflammation in the brain and the tumor causes inflammation as it dies. But we are past the acute phase."

Although I'm afraid of more seizures, I try to keep my mind open and believe what Dr. Engle is saying. "I'm concerned about breakthrough pain. I feel we need something at home for quick-acting pain relief."

"We will give Jack a prescription for pain meds." Dr. Engle shifts his gaze to Jack. "I want you to dial down on the pain meds, to lighten up on them, as soon as you are able. I have you on the maximum treatment you can handle right now and we are in the waiting phase. I am cautiously optimistic. When areas heal we are going forward with your chemo as scheduled."

Dr. Engle explains a few details of checking into the clinic for Jack's next chemo, and before he leaves, he makes eye contact with us both. "You should call Hospice and get enrolled as soon as you get home."

CHAPTER 11

Managing As An Outpatient

Wednesday, January 18 – Monday, January 30

Living at home again doesn't just shift us back where we were. Nothing is the same. Managing Jack's care as a cancer outpatient brings with it a whole new set of feelings and challenges. Some I'm ready for but others I just keep fighting to control.

Nursing

Being a decent caregiver starts with managing meds. I make charts to record when and what meds to give Jack. The charts aren't clear enough for me so I make tables instead. I send Conrad to buy two thermometers, a blood pressure cuff and pill dispensers at CVS – both simple and complex models. I set up temporary shelves on the counter in our bathroom and organize Jack's meds onto three shelves – top shelf for those he takes more than once a day, middle shelf for the ones he takes once a day, bottom shelf for the meds he takes "as needed." I remake my med-recording tables because the first one doesn't include lines to keep track of Jack's vitals. I want to record them in the same place I check off his meds. No matter what I do, I fret that I will either under or over dose Jack.

Families function differently with roles and relationships formed by the individuals within the family. I know that within the larger Rankie family, my Shelton family has, over the years, undergone close scrutiny and sometimes, strong negative criticism. My placement as the youngest sibling and Conrad's as the only only-child in his generation of Rankies open us up to less-respected roles. Conrad has been judged with expectations for him, and his level of responsibility is almost constantly questioned. When Conrad was a very young child my father once said to Jack and me, "You let the tail wag the dog." I had to ask Jack to explain what my father meant, but after that I started to understand the different comments my family made and didn't need Jack's translation. I've tried to forget and forgive but some of the comments are burned in my mind because they were made more than once. Things like, "Well, you can do things differently because you only have one child." Or "When you have more than one child you have to say 'No' to your kids once in a while." And "Nancy, you'll learn. Just give yourself time."

Regardless of the repeated messages that Jack and I are inferior parents and I am not old enough to know what I'm doing, I know I'm a good parent and an intelligent, successful, professional woman. I also know in my heart that as Kiley, Conrad, Jack and I negotiate our way through this traumatic experience that it's inevitable I will again feel disapproval projected towards Conrad. Now that I'm home and will start seeing and talking to family more often, I mentally and emotionally brace myself for the kinds of unspoken messages about my son that will inevitably be sent my way.

Conrad has been involved in Jack's struggle in the most helpful ways possible. He and Kiley have been doing our laundry, delivering food, books and the newspaper, and completing any other chores that would demand time or energy from us that we cannot give. They have visited us as much as we want them to visit. It is in the visiting that Conrad has perceived more than anything else what Jack and I need.

When Jack was in the hospital, he didn't want Conrad hanging around all the time. Jack's own memories of his father suffering from scleroderma have haunted Jack his whole life. He simply refuses to pass that legacy to Conrad. But now at home where we are coping with recovery, Conrad's role is becoming more substantial every day. Matt is back to continue physical therapy and the occupational therapist is also on board. Conrad works with Jack for all his exercises and when they work out, I sink into the bathtub. Conrad has become my back-up nurse, helping me with every aspect of Jack's care.

Transportation

Jack's outpatient radiation is scheduled for consecutive weekdays for the next 19 days, so even though we just got home I have to drive Jack back to Shands. Mentally I rehearse the trip, allowing for extra time for Jack to get in and out of the car. We have valet parking passes from the clinic so I know the drive and parking won't take that much longer than normal. I also don't want to be too early because I don't want Jack sitting in a germ-filled environment very long waiting for his treatment.

Jack's wheelchair is the small, lighter version, but it's still heavy and with moving wheels, it's awkward to maneuver into my trunk. Clearly I have relied too heavily on Jack for many years because now that I'm responsible for all the heavy lifting I see I'm not as strong as I once was. Well, that will change. It starts to rain as we approach Shands. It's just a light rain but still, it's one more obstacle.

"Where are you going to park?" Jack asks. Steve was right, Jack's speech is better every day and he sounds like himself again, but his words still come slowly.

"They gave us valet parking passes, I'm going to use one of those."

"No. I don't want to leave our car with the valet. They don't drive it carefully enough."

"Well I was planning to use it. Are you sure we can't? Just this once?"

"I don't want someone raising hell with this car." Though Jack bought the car for me, he's damn proud of it and very protective.

We get to the parking area and I have to drive around to the outside edges to find a space where there's enough room to fully open the door so I can help Jack transfer from the car to the wheelchair. I finally find one I think is spacious enough and pull in.

Leaving Jack in the passenger seat, I hurry to the trunk and get the wheelchair out, wheel it to Jack's door and try to position the chair. There's not enough room.

"Why don't you just pull half-way out of the spot and let me get out, then park the car."

Damn, I think, *he's still got a sharper mind with more solutions than I.*

As I begin pushing Jack to the building, I start a mental "inventory" to make sure I have everything we need. *We're on time. I know where I've parked the car. Jack has his cap and jacket. Do I have Jack's wallet and the check-in IMPAC card he needs for his radiation?* "Oh no. Jack, I forgot my purse. I'll be right back. I'll just run back and grab it."

I turn and run back to the car, grab my purse, and frantically head back through the parking lot to where I left Jack. I look up and see Jack in his wheelchair and I realize what I've done – I left my husband stranded, in the rain, in a wheelchair, in the middle of the parking lot. He has no way to get out of the way of an oncoming car, no way to get out of the rain, no way to protect himself.

Oh my God… I have a lot to learn.

Staying upright

Even before Jack's seizure, life in the Shelton house was influenced by illness. Kiley has not been feeling well and she's tried a number of strategies, including changing her diet, to help. But she never complains to me and I wouldn't know she's even sick if Conrad didn't tell me. I wish I could do more for her and ask less from her, but I have no way to survive any other way than the way I am managing each day.

When I see how Kiley and Conrad have transformed my study into a great space for Jack and me to relax, the gratitude I feel is overwhelming. We have a new 3-D television set on a modern, glass TV table. The couch they moved into the room is just the right height to allow Jack to get up and down pretty easily, and there's plenty of floor space for the wheelchair. Our third night home Jack and I decide to watch a movie together. Kiley and Conrad have gone out and we are home alone for the first time since Terrible Tuesday.

Jack needs to relieve himself and I'm not sure I can manage getting him into the bathroom. So I decide it will be better to move the portable toilet to the couch – there's room enough and I think it will be easier than helping Jack maneuver into the bathroom.

I set the chair up at an angle I think will allow Jack to just stand, pivot, and sit on the portable toilet. Seems simple enough…

Jack stands. He starts to pivot. He leans towards me. In seconds we crash to the floor. My mouth and Jack's head simultaneously smash into the glass TV table. My knee and my back absorb the shock from Jack's and my weight slamming onto the floor. My arms are pinned under me and Jack lands on top of me.

"Holy shit." I manage. "Are you okay?"

"Better question – are you okay?"

The two of us just lay on the floor laughing. It's an explosion of relief. We laugh at our stupidity. We laugh because neither one of us can get up. We laugh at the absolute insanity that our lives have become.

Jack's hand slammed against the table, or the TV (who knows which), and blood pools under his nail. Thank God he didn't suffer significant damage because we aren't telling anyone that we fell.

We don't share details of how he smashed his finger. It's our secret. Nothing else about Jack's body is private but we still manage to smile at something no one else knows.

Catching up

My father is celebrating his 85th birthday. Jack and I had planned a trip to Sun City Center, where we were going to surprise my parents by arranging a dinner with my siblings John and Jeanne. But, since Terrible Tuesday, we've all made adjustments to our plans. John already came down earlier this month, but Jeanne is in Florida now.

She and her friend, Andre, make the drive from the Tampa area to visit us. It's good to see family. It's the first time Jeanne has been to our house in Florida. It's nice to show her around.

While Jeanne and Andre are here, Sue calls and asks if she and Dale can come to visit. Sue has wanted to come up from Crystal River to see Jack since he had the seizure, but there just hasn't been an opportunity. Jack has seen Pat and Kelly and I know he wants to visit with Sue. Sue and Dale have been married for a few years and he and Jack get along well.

When I ask Jack if he's up for additional visitors, Jeanne offers to leave so that Jack can visit with Sue and Dale, but Jack asks her to stay. Andre and Jeanne have lunch with us and shortly after we finish eating Sue and Dale arrive. When Andre and Jeanne head back to my parents it's difficult to say goodbye. As Jeanne and I embrace, though I don't say it, I wonder if Jeanne will ever see Jack again. I think she's wondering the same thing.

It's a long day for Jack. He's visibly getting weaker as the visiting continues. Miraculously, his hiccups have been gone for two days, but they come back early this afternoon. That's a bad sign. I'm worried Jack is stressing himself too much. I have to ask Sue and Dale to go so Jack can take a nap.

Kiley has been traveling frequently to her parents' home in the

Florida Panhandle. Jack and I make a point of trying our best not to ask too many questions or interfere with Conrad and Kiley's personal business, and we didn't have a plan to gather for Christmas. We were letting things "fall into place" in a way that could accommodate us all.

Now, with Jack's cancer front and center, we need to plan. Jack has been out of the hospital for a week and Kiley's parents, Mike and Kathy, come to visit. Kiley is very close to her parents, and though I'm sure they are concerned about Jack, it's most likely that they want to help Kiley manage her stress and sadness. At times like this, normal chores like shopping, house cleaning and maintenance fall by the wayside. Mike and Kathy just set out to help, scrubbing walls, cleaning floors, cooking, baking and preparing a delayed Christmas celebration.

Foundational help

Many of our friends and family have asked, "What can we do for you?" and said, "How can we help – just let us know and we're there for you." But I honestly can't say what I need, either because I can't recognize what I need or because I just can't ask.

A few people don't ask, they just do. I wonder every day why this is and hope that I, while just trying to hold on to the little bit of strength I feel inside, am not offending anyone who I care about and who cares about me. Len and Morna are a great example. They are getting the construction in our family room done as much as they can before we head back to Maryland. They live close enough to our home in Maryland that when I need anything (e.g. Jack's will dug out of my file cabinet and sent to us, our title for the SUV we traded in located and mailed to the dealership, my plants watered) Morna just does it. But I rarely call her and update her on Jack's condition. I don't send emails unless I need help. I give nothing in return for the favors I ask.

And Bess, my research partner and wife of Jack's neurologist, plays a different role. She is constantly by my side even though she's hundreds of miles away. She has medical knowledge she shares when asked (and not before), can help me juggle issues surrounding my job, and is taking the lead role in communicating to our publisher and other research partners about the project we've been working on for the past three years. She seems to understand on an unspoken level what I am feeling. Her compassion is comforting in a way that I can't describe. And though we didn't get Shands to send Jack's records to Steve as he suggested during our phone conversation, I know that as soon as we get back to Maryland Jack and I will be visiting Steve at his office.

And there are other friends – too many to name – who have helped us adjust to this "new normal" in multiple ways. I've become comfortable with the dynamics in my friendships and know that the passage of time will be the final test of strength in the relationships. It's not been so easy with the undercurrents involved in family ties. I make a note:

Compassion

Compassion knocks on my door. I stare through the two-inch crack. Indifferent to the tenderness etched in her face.

"Nancy, I was in your neighborhood and thought I'd see if you had time for a cup of tea." Her confidence offered as comfort.

Yea right. I think. *An innocent cup of tea. I don't think so.*

Compassion just waits. Quiet. Eyes full of kindness and patience.

I had better answer something or else she'll never leave me alone.

"Well, thanks," I force. "I appreciate it. I really I do. But it's not a good time. Another time, maybe."

"No problem, Nancy. It's okay if you're not ready to invite me in. I'll patiently wait out here on your porch. When you've satiated yourself with grief, anger and self-pity, I'll be here for you."

From this journey's onset I've told my family, the Rankies, that I'm unable to communicate on any kind of schedule, and that I will be in touch when possible. When asked if I want anyone in my family to come help, I say, "It's okay, we're managing."

My sister Carol and my brother John refused to take this as an answer. When they came to visit on January 10, as soon as I saw them I knew that I needed their help. But I can't ask for it. I can't sit and think what I need from other people. I don't have the emotional energy to be disappointed by an unanswered request, or an off-handed, and I am sure sincere, offer to "be there for us" that just isn't going to happen. I don't have the energy to put into the esoteric "what do I need" as opposed to just finding the energy within myself to meet each challenge as it presents itself.

Not crying

When I was a child, my mother taught me that you never cry in public. If I couldn't handle my emotions, my mother sent me to my bedroom to do my crying privately.

As an adult, I know crying is culturally bound, that it helps some people and not others, and that the conditions that cause a person to cry often impact the emotional value of crying. I also know myself and have figured out well before Terrible Tuesday what benefits crying have in my life.

Whether or not it's because of my mother or the fact that in my job as a teacher of both young children and college students I have sat with more students crying than I care to count, I prefer to cry alone. I don't typically cry over happy occasions. Sometimes tears leak out of my eyes when someone says something insulting to me, but that's not really crying in my book. When I cry it's usually a fierce release of emotion. I'll isolate myself, have a wicked, loud, sobbing wail, and then clean up and get on with life.

I feel every bit of the fear, anguish, sadness, and terror that has entered my life. I know I need some way to release my emotions. But I can't cry. I dare not chance letting my grief express itself. Small bouts of relief are necessary, and when I know I can't go another hour without letting some measure of tension escape in order to make room for more that I know will develop, I call one of the three people with whom I have made an agreement – Carol, Bess and Morna. "No words necessary," they have said, "You can just cry if that's what you need." They see my number in their caller ID and I don't even have to speak. I often don't.

But even these sessions have to be brief and controlled. Something in me knows I can't really let go. If I do, I may never get back. I can't cry in front of Jack. I can't let him witness my fright. I can't let him feel my anxiety.

Shenanigans

As Jack gets stronger and is able to move in his wheelchair, I feel more able to leave the house and venture off to places I need to go. I've gotten a haircut, been shopping at Publix and gone to CVS to fill Jack's prescriptions.

Jack and Conrad manage well together. They don't smother each other with attention, but are available when either needs something.

Conrad and I have shifted into a comfortable shared care for Jack. Knowing we can't leave him alone, we give each other time to do what we need to do to be out of the house. If I'm uncomfortable going on an errand, Conrad asks no questions – he just does what I need.

"Mom, here's Dad's meds. I'll put them on the counter in your bathroom."

As I walk into the bathroom I notice Conrad is walking toward Jack with another bag. I stop ruffling the prescription bags so I can hear what they say to each other. I don't want to intrude, but I am curious.

"Dad, I got you something."

"Thanks Kid. What is it?"

"Just look in the bag."

"What? A pair of handcuffs? What's this for?"

"That's so you don't lose your wheelchair if you keep up your shenanigans. I'm going to cuff you to your chair."

Father and son laugh together as they explain. Yesterday Conrad was walking from the kitchen to his bedroom and he glanced down the hall to see Jack lying on the floor, his wheelchair several feet away.

"Dad – what are you doing?" Conrad had asked.

"Oh, I just thought I could reach something but found out I couldn't when I tipped my chair over. Now I'm trying to reach the chair."

In typical Shelton fashion, Conrad has turned a serious situation into something to keep us smiling, and while doing so, blessed us with a new Shelton family saying – "No more shenanigans."

Panic attacks

The first was the worst. We are in bed, sleeping, when Jack bolts into a sitting position and just keeps saying "No! No! No!" Over and over again.

He can't tell me what's wrong. He can't say anything more than "No." And though he thrashes around, he can't get out of bed.

That night, and every night since then, I hold him. I stroke his hair, rub his back, and hold him as tightly as I can. Eventually he calms down, but even then he can't say what strikes the panic in him.

Jack has become afraid of the dark. We keep two or three candles lit – one in the bathroom, one beside our bed, and one on the dresser.

The physicians say Decadron can cause these attacks, but we can't lower the dose because if we do, we increase the chance of another seizure.

So every night, panic comes to us as regularly as the setting sun.

Follow up appointments

I think I know Gainesville. But I forget that Gainesville changes and grows while I'm in Maryland teaching. Though we come back for at least two months every year, I'm beginning to realize that I only know parts of Gainesville. This realization comes when I make a mistake, which I have done.

It's Monday, January 23. Finally we get to go to see Dr. Oliver, Jack's orthopedic surgeon. We've been looking forward to this day since Jack's initial confinement to the wheelchair. His hip has been radiated for seven days and Jack is no longer in pain. This afternoon Jack will go for his eighth hip and his fifth lung XRT. We just need a "green light" so that Jack can start weight-bearing physical therapy and get back on his feet more than just to pivot from the chair to the car, or the chair to the toilet.

We arrive at Shands Plaza on Archer Road, unload Jack, and start searching for the correct office. Very soon I become completely confused, pull out my cell phone, and call the number on Jack's appointment card.

"Hull Road?" I say. "Oh my gosh, I've taken Jack to the wrong office."

The receptionist is amused. I hear her chuckle. "It's okay Mrs. Shelton. We'll hold Mr. Shelton's appointment for him."

Feeling harried I'm delighted to be greeted by Trey once we're finally in the examining room. His cheery demeanor persists as we joke about how great it is to see him when Jack and I are fully dressed, it's not 7:00 AM, and we're not at the hospital.

However, our chipper attitude lasts only so long. Trey examines

Jack's scans and delivers the bad news. It's too risky for Jack to put weight on his damaged hip.

I'm devastated.

Jack is mute.

"The problem is we have no recourse if you were to fall or in any way damage the joint."

Jack and I remain voiceless.

"You will see Dr. Oliver next. I'll go tell him you are ready."

Jack and I sit in the cold, sterile examining room waiting. I feel the simultaneous urge to speak and to be silent. I give respect to silence.

The door opens. Dr. Oliver is a handsome man. Normally that would be of comfort to me but this morning it's insignificant. He smiles as he sits on the little black stool on wheels. He rolls over to face Jack. I'm beside Jack, sitting on the chair typically intended for the patient.

"Mr. Shelton, it's good to see you," he begins. "I have good news. Although I want you to be careful, you can start physical therapy and become fully-weight bearing again."

"But Trey just said it was too risky," Jack comments.

"No, the area damaged is on the very tip of your acetabulum and it's protected enough that if you're careful, you should be okay. But I don't want you out there playing tennis."

Within minutes we are given a follow-up appointment and dismissed for the day.

Once in the elevator I say, "Oh my God Jack, I thought you weren't going to be able to get back on your feet."

The office was only on the third floor and I'm pushing Jack through the building's exterior doors by the time he answers me. "I know. I really like Trey but I am glad he was wrong."

"I have to scream. I have to let it out. Scream with me Jack."

"No, Nancy. I'm not screaming."

"Well I am."

"Go ahead – knock yourself out."

Jack knows I *hate* that expression so just to be a jerk back at him I start running, pushing him as I go, screaming wildly as I cross through two parking lots.

I finally calm down when I get to the car where I see a parking ticket on our windshield. In my haste to get to the correct address I didn't carefully read the signs and had parked in the employee lot. I was just looking for a parking space with vacant spaces around it so I could park and get Jack out of the car. I refuse to let the ticket squelch my happiness. Dr. Oliver just gave me the documentation I need to get special parking so I won't have to struggle getting Jack in and out of the car any more. Besides that, Jack will soon be walking again.

I'm not accustomed to going out for more than one task, and realize that while we have time for lunch, we have no lunch. Conrad has no hesitation when I ask him to go by a deli and pick lunch up for us, and deliver it to the picnic tables outside the plaza where Jack is being treated. We have lunch together in the sunshine. After Jack's XRT I drive directly to the Motor Vehicle Department, leave Jack in the car, and get the handicap hangtag. By the time we get home Jack is completely exhausted, so I tuck him in for a nap. I pick up my laptop and write a letter to the University of Florida police requesting that they excuse my ticket. I feel so good I'm sure they will comply.

Having made it through the first follow-up appointment I'm better prepared to get Jack to the neurology office to see Dr. Hoffman. For this I have a list of questions, most important is to ask about Jack's nighttime panic attacks. Dr. Hoffman provides us with a schedule to gradually decrease Jack's Decadron to see if that will help him sleep through the night. He also prescribes Ativan for Jack to help when he has an anxiety attack and Ambien to use to help him sleep. Although Jack prefers not to load his body with drugs, he understands that these panic attacks need to be treated.

Jack's partial seizures were on the cusp of becoming generalized, which is not a good thing, so Dr. Hoffman increased Jack's anti-seizure meds. Again we're assured that Jack's postictal changes (lethargy and limb paralysis) will continue to improve.

Daily routine

Every morning as soon as we wake I take Jack's temperature and give him his meds. I wash him and dress him, wash myself and dress, and then if it's a day when Matt is coming for PT I rush Jack's breakfast (two pieces of toast and jam). Then I sit and have coffee or take a hot bath while Conrad, Matt and Jack work on Jack's PT. We go to XRT every weekday about 11 am.

If it's not a day when Matt comes for PT we have coffee, discuss the news and then we shower. Shower days are an ordeal but after a couple of hours, we are dressed and ready for XRT so I load Jack up and drive to Shands (the Davis Cancer Center) where we check in, get the XRT done and hopefully get back home without having to spend too much time waiting for this or that doctor or procedure. When we are at Shands moving from one office to the next, seeing specialists, checking in with the Radiation Oncologist or seeing the Medical Oncologist I don't have one ounce of energy for the rest of the day.

Jack is completely out of pain from his hip, but he can't get rid of the damn hiccups, which go on for *hours* day after day and hurt him physically and emotionally.

We've also learned that the MRIs show that Jack has the same three brain tumors, that they haven't changed in size, and that it takes three months for the radiation to affect the DNA of the tumors. We also now know that Jack's cancer doesn't have the mutation we had hoped for, but we also expected this because the mutation is concentrated in patients who are nonsmokers. and Jack was a smoker. We've started to understand all the tests that need to be done before chemo – they were done when Jack was an inpatient, but we just didn't know exactly what all the blood work was testing for. The port Jack has helps – at least his arm isn't doubling as a pincushion.

I often think about people who are not as fortunate as Jack and I are in terms of being granted family or sick leave from employment. What do they do when cancer takes over their lives? I'm glad Jack and I have professional careers. I feel sad for others who don't.

It's a full time job getting to all the medical appointments. As exhausting as it is for me, I'm at least full-strength. Jack is moving more and more slowly, trying to keep his weight up. But he's struggling. He's drinking a gallon of water a day and takes regular naps. Both will help him keep strong and build back some of what he has lost.

Jack and I are constantly worried about how his cancer is affecting Kiley and Conrad. Kiley has been feeling poorly. She's not her usual cheerful self. I'm sure a lot of it is because of the stress she feels with us being here and with Jack's illness. Conrad has taken time off work, which must be difficult for them. I've assured Conrad that I can manage if he goes back to work, but in truth I know I need him. He takes care of the shopping, the laundry, the house and the dogs. When Jack had to face the fact that his hair was falling out in chunks, it was to Conrad he turned, not me.

But most importantly, Conrad is Jack's physical therapy assistant. He stays with Matt and Jack observing everything Jack does during his therapy. On Matt's off days, Conrad does all Jack's exercises with him at least twice a day. Since I can't hold Jack up if he falls, Jack needs Conrad to learn to walk again. Watching Conrad hold onto the belt around Jack and stay with him every inch of the way across the kitchen and down the hall is an encouraging sight for me.

Jack now has all the stigmata of cancer. Always conscious of his physique and proud of his broad shoulders and slim hips, he's quickly become just plain skinny. Always quick on his feet, he's now wheelchair bound. Although my father has teased Jack since he was in his early thirties, pointing out that Jack's receding hairline was advancing much more quickly than his father-in-law's, Jack is now bald.

CHAPTER 12

Five More Days At Shands

Tuesday, January 31

We're back at Shands.

Yesterday afternoon Jack and Conrad watched Harry Potter in 3-D on the new TV. They looked like teenagers wearing their 3-D glasses, laughing and dodging flying objects that would never leave the television screen.

Jack's language is back, he moves his hand and arm more and more every day, and he's able to walk with a cane for short distances. Laughter re-entered our lives.

We gathered for dinner, sitting around the table in what felt like an almost-normal Shelton meal. After just a few minutes I noticed Jack wasn't eating. I hesitated to say anything because I wasn't sure if he just felt awkward or if something was wrong.

Too much time passed with Jack not talking, not eating.

"Are you okay, Honey?"

"My chest is starting to hurt. I'll be okay. I just need to slow down."

Hoping Jack's self-assessment was accurate, we all continued eating.

Suddenly, Jack let out a little scream and grabbed his chest. "What is it Jack? What's wrong?"

I made eye contact with Conrad. Fear was etched on his face.

"Dad, can I get you something? Do you want to go lie down?"

Jack could barely respond. His breathing was short, labored, making it obvious he was in great pain. He was leaning forward, clutching his chest. Between breaths and painful grunts Jack managed to say, "I don't know what it is son, but you better call 911. It's getting worse and it's in my chest. Not only do I hurt, I can't take a chance with chest pain."

After another night in the ER Jack was moved to the fifth floor even though we requested, no, *insisted*, that he needed to be on 8 East. Apparently the doctors in the ER have total power over where a patient is transferred, so now I have to work to get Jack back where he belongs. We've notified both Drs. Engle and Tran. At noon Dr. Tran comes down to see Jack. He promises us that he will get Jack transferred to the 8 East oncology floor.

Jack's pain, which has been constant for several hours, is serious. Just after noon they give him a Dilaudid pump. Dilaudid is an opioid analgesic and can have serious side effects. The increase in prescriptions for drugs that are heavily controlled because they can lead to addictive dependence concerns me, but I don't say anything to anyone. The bottom line is that Jack needs something to relieve the pain.

They already did a CT and have ordered an ECHO of his heart. It's complicated to treat Jack – they are concerned the pain is caused by a blood clot, but Heparin, which is what they would normally prescribe for a clot, is dangerous because of Jack's brain mets.

Throughout the day a constant flow of professionals examine Jack. There's no doubt about it, these doctors don't mess around when they are concerned about heart involvement. Their first suspicion is that Jack may have a pulmonary embolism, but they've tested for heart attack, pericarditis, aortic dissection, and pneumonia (and post obstructive pneumonia). By 2:00 PM they conclude that whatever is causing the pain isn't pulmonary and are willing to let the oncologists take over decision-making.

Wednesday, February 1

It's been decided that Jack will continue his XRT while here. Gratefully, we're back in the world of 8 East, where there's nothing unfamiliar in the odors, the sounds, the stored equipment in the corridor, the carts that hold sheets and towels, and the various machines' flashing digitized lights. I've come to know the machines, what they are for, how they work, whether or not we might need them for Jack. Walking around the hospital is as normal as taking a walk around the block in our neighborhood, something we often did when Juno was a puppy.

Dr. Norman is on rounds. It's the first I have seen him in many years. I was a caregiver for two children, grandsons to one of Norman's patients. I frequently brought the children to the hospital to visit their grandfather, and more often I visited without the children. On those occasions I saw Dr. Norman many times and had passing conversations with him. He doesn't remember me but I remember him. I suppose it's very much that way for us all – the physician is more of an individual to a patient and the patient's family than the patient is to the physician.

Dr. Norman explains that Jack's white blood cell count is very low. The lowest point is usually six days after chemo. Since Jack's next infusion is scheduled tomorrow, they will keep a watch on Jack's blood cell counts. Dr. Norman thinks Jack's pain is caused by an irritation of the nerves in the pleura, which is the outer layer of the lung. There are no nerves in the lung, but there is something called referred pain, which is pain that is being caused in one area of the body but felt in another. He conjectures that the radiation to the mass in the back of Jack's lung could have irritated a nerve. He implies that the only permanent fix for the pain is to continue radiation and further minimize the mass.

Jack is getting regular shots of Heparin subcutaneously to prevent blood clotting. His belly is starting to look like one huge bruise.

Thursday, February 2

The role that the nurses play in Jack's care is essential. Madison has come to visit Jack on more than one occasion. She is one of Jack's nurses who is always smiling and always willing to make a difficult situation seem normal.

"Mr. Shelton. You just like us too much. You can't seem to stay away."

"Oh Madison, I'd like to stay away. But you know what I have been saying – *The hits just keep on coming.*"

As I watch the interaction between Jack and Madison, I run video after video of life through my mind trying to find a comparison, a precedent, an explanation. Jack has been constipated. He doesn't talk about it. He doesn't complain of discomfort. But Madison knows and she offers him relief. The topic is as natural as one about the weather. "Well, let me take care of you. I'm known as the best 'Hinny Nurse' in the hospital and while we're making you feel better, I'm going to help you with a shower."

I quietly observe. Madison is perfect – the exact professional, kind person who Jack needs at this moment. Jack and Madison continue talking and I feel like my presence in the room is insignificant. I could leave and it wouldn't matter. Though I desperately need a break, I don't want to relinquish the intimacy I have owned for decades, even if it is to a nurse who clearly needs to take the role she's taking. She's done it with such skill that Jack is willing to let her. He's going to accept the suppository, which I know is what he needs so I tell my emotions to behave. She's going to give Jack a shower.

Heated towels. Efficient movements. Madison has commanded what needs to be done. I'm able to relax. To sit and watch. To think about nothing except that Jack is contentedly taking a shower. My muscles start to feel relief from the fatigue that has gripped me to the core. I can feel tension escaping my body. The voices I hear are pleasant, even congenial. I start to wonder if I'm finally escaping from this hell I've been living in when suddenly Madison pulls me back to reality.

Her voice has raised a few decibels and is cheerful. I realize she's no longer talking to Jack but to me. "Be sure to put towels around the bathroom floor and don't use them sparingly, use what you need. Be sure to always get Jack heated towels so that when he turns the water off he doesn't get cold. And I can't tell you what else to do, you know as his wife he needs your warm touch."

Oh my god, I think, *she knows what I've been thinking. She knows I need to be honored as Jack's wife while still being shown how to best help him. She is as important as the doctors.*

After Jack is situated back in bed, he's hooked up to the infusion machine and his chemo is started.

Friday, February 3

Today is an observation day. Other than physical and occupational therapy, the goal for Jack's care is to transition him from Dilaudid to Morphine so we can get back home. Jack has asked to be discharged – nothing at the hospital is adding to his recovery and he'd rather be home than at Shands. The facts at this point are:

1. The pain is intense and near the lesion in Jack's lung.
2. The doctors don't know what is causing the pain.
3. Jack's heart again tested well – it's not the problem.
4. They have found no clots or embolisms.
5. Jack continues to have panic/anxiety attacks, but now they include pain.

There are several theories for the attacks – again more conjectures or possibilities than facts:

1. One of the drugs, Decadron, is known to cause psychosis and other psychotic episodes as a side effect. Jack is tapering from the drug and has just two more days to be on it.

2. Brain radiation can cause day/night confusion in some patients. I doubt this is the cause because Jack's brain surgery was well before the attacks.

3. Any number of the drugs and/or interactions between the multitude of drugs (especially the anti-seizure drugs) can cause lack of sleep and anxiety.

4. The diagnosis and seriousness of Jack's disease can cause physiological stress.

Whatever the reason, because he can't sleep at night, Jack sleeps most of the day. I spend the day answering emails about my job, reading, and taking care of home-related business. Jack and I had intended to stay in Florida until the last week in January, so all our bills are paid and the mail was stopped until then. But it's February, and I need to make sure our cat, bills, and plants are all taken care of until we can get back to Maryland.

Mikey, a former student and now our friend, is going to change the mailbox and install a larger box so that our mail isn't exposed to the elements. Katie, another former student-now-friend, and her husband Jake, have given our cat, Hei Mei, a home. Katie has also volunteered to drive by the house once a week and send all the collected mail to us in a priority mailer. Len and Morna will keep working on the family room walls as much as time allows.

Saturday, February 4

Early this morning Dr. Engle comes by to let us know he's approved discharge for Jack. The follow up care Jack needs includes a Complete Blood Count (CBC), which can be done through the Shands Family Practice system. Once again Dr. Engle emphasizes that Jack needs to sign up for Hospice Care.

At 3:15 PM Jack is discharged. We head home.

CHAPTER 13

Getting Back On Our Feet

February 5 – February 29

Each semester I teach at the university I provide a tentative schedule that outlines the course for my students. I always introduce the schedule as *tentative* and emphasize that the students should expect changes, not work or look too far ahead, and be flexible to the adjustments that will need to be made. Tentative. That's the best word to describe our lives. We proceed with caution, knowing that changes are likely to erupt without warning.

Hospice

When we first heard the word *Hospice*, strong rejection rose in us. But after four emergency admittances to Shands and feeling pure fatigue, we know it's time. I need help and Jack needs care for issues too trite for oncologists.

Conrad can't emotionally handle this. Whenever we talk about Hospice, he leaves the room. Jack and I notice this, and don't talk about it in front of him. We let him know in advance we have sched-uled an appointment so that if he wants, he can leave the house.

In Alachua County, there's just one Hospice provider, *Haven*

Hospice. On February 7 the administrative nurse, Faye, comes to our home and Jack signs the papers to be admitted into the program.

Jack's providers will be *Team A.* Besides providing nursing care, *Haven* has doctors who will make house calls, social workers and volunteers. We work out the frequency of home visits Jack's nurse will make based on our needs.

A group called "Palliative Care" joined with Hospice and together they are experts in symptom management. They work hard to break down a patient's symptoms to adjust medications so that the patient is in the absolute greatest possible comfort.

The Hospice doctor only manages symptoms, and Dr. Engle is still Jack's primary oncologist. If Jack's symptoms (pain, nausea, breathing difficulties) get out of control, we can call Hospice first. If it's necessary to go back to Shands, the Hospice Hospital Team will work with us there.

Faye presents us with two folders full of information and documentation.

When we meet Lisa, Team A Social Worker, and Cheryl, Jack's nurse, I'm still uncomfortable, and feel like Hospice is an intervention I'm not sure I want. Lisa has to "inspect" our house. That is easy – everything is set up for Jack and she has nothing to suggest.

Cheryl needs to go over all of Jack's meds, how often they are given, what his schedule is like, his diet, and his general health beyond his cancer diagnosis. When I show her the temporary shelves I set up in our bathroom, she takes two of the meds off the shelf and writes on the labels.

I hide my anger. I'm a writing teacher. I teach my students that you *never* write on another writer's paper without prior permission. It's an issue of ownership. Cheryl has just violated my ownership of Jack's care. I resent her and her intrusion.

Jack can hear that my voice is strained and takes over all conversation with Cheryl and Lisa. I try to control my tone, but it's something I have struggled with my whole life. When I am angry it shows.

"Look at this, Jack," I say as I hand Jack the Ambien and Ativan to show him how Cheryl had written on them.

"Relax, Nancy. She's just doing her job. She didn't mean to insult you. They are both nice women."

I know Jack is right. I turn the bottles so her handwriting isn't visible to me. When I take a minute to think about my anger, I know that it's true – I don't like someone coming into my house and claiming possession of my organization system, but the deeper source of my anger is Jack's cancer coming into our lives and taking all control away from us.

Outpatient clinic

It has taken more weeks than we expected for Jack to become an outpatient chemo patient. It's another "first" I would prefer not to experience.

The waiting rooms at Dr. Engle's clinic/office are huge. I've never seen so many people who have cancer gathered in one place. I survey the room and am overwhelmed by the obvious evidence of illness stamped on just about every person around us.

Our first visit on February 8 is for Jack to meet the staff, have lab work completed, and for us to become familiar with the facility. Janese is Dr. Engle's assistant, and we will work more closely with her than Dr. Engle.

After all the medical issues are addressed, we're directed to the social worker's office at Dr. Engle's clinic to let her know we've signed up for Hospice and to get Jack's FMLA (family leave) papers completed. Since we didn't call ahead, we have to wait to see her.

She finally calls us into her office. It's hard for me to maneuver Jack's wheelchair in, but I manage. The only space for him is the most distant point from the social worker's desk. Once he's situated, I sit in the chair next to the desk.

"Good morning," I begin. "Thank you for seeing us."

The social worker looks at Jack, not me, and with no greeting to either of us asks, "How can I help you, Mr. Shelton?"

"Dr. Engle encouraged us to sign up for Hospice –" I try to explain, hoping my voice doesn't crack.

She abruptly interrupts me. "Mr. Shelton, is there a reason you are here this morning?"

Jack just looks at me. It's obvious that neither of us expected this woman's abruptness. I try again. "I was saying that Dr. Engle –"

"Yes, I know what you were saying. I was asking Mr. Shelton a question."

I look at Jack. "This isn't working honey. Let's go."

"Okay." His eyes tell me more than that single word. He knows this woman is being rude. It's hard enough for us to go through this, and we don't need additional frustration.

In his usual steadiness, Jack responds to the social worker. "My wife and I will come back another time. Thank you." I start to gather my belongings so I can maneuver Jack's wheelchair back out of the office and escape from this hostile environment.

"Oh. I'm sorry. Are you sure I can't help you with something?" she says in a voice that doesn't reveal whether or not she realizes her disrespect and offensiveness.

I'm very direct but maintain a civil tone. "We're here because Dr. Engle said you would help us with the FMLA papers. But if you can't let me talk, it's better that we come back another time."

My candor was effective. She finally softens slightly and says, "I am sorry. I've had a rough morning. I apologize. I'll be glad to help you."

I can't stop tears from forming, my nose fills with mucous, my throat constricts and I can't talk because I'll just shift into a full cry. I stop pushing my notebook back into my bag, concentrate on breathing to calm myself, blink a few times to stop the blurring in my vision, and look at Jack. I realize I need to make this conversation happen.

An hour later, with FMLA papers in hand, additional information about the need to immediately register for Social Security Disability, and an appointment card for our next visit, we escape.

"Gosh – can you believe that woman is a social worker?" I ask Jack.

"She sure forgot her profession there for a while, didn't she? I thought you handled yourself well though. I'm glad she got it together and we got this business done. We didn't know anything at all about Social Security Disability benefits. We'll have to follow up on that right away."

As I walk to the parking lot, pushing Jack, my tears come back. How am I going to manage to love myself when I don't have Jack to let me know I'm an okay person? That woman was vicious. I could just as easily have been a bitch back at her but I wasn't. And a big reason I wasn't is that I'm a better person when I'm with Jack. It feels good to know that he recognizes my efforts and is proud of me. How will I be able to feel that when this cancer steals him from me?

Touch

One hot, summer afternoon in 1977 just after Jack and I had met, we were walking down 8th Avenue in Pass-A-Grille Beach when I reached out to hold Jack's hand. Jack looked at me and calmly said, "I am not the hand-holding type." Shocked, I yanked my hand back to my side and put a little distance between us as we walked.

Time passed and he found comfort in being touched. Even with the special physical ease we now share, we don't really hold hands. We lock a few fingers – Jack's pointer and middle finger with my ring finger and pinky. It's just a loose weave but one that's strong enough to hold us together.

As I'm sure happens with other couples, Jack and I have developed other rituals of tenderness. Every night when we're lying in bed, just before we fall asleep we each extend one foot towards the other. Jack sleeps on his back and I sleep on my stomach so my right foot is always snuggled in the arch of Jack's right foot. We don't stay like this all night and we share many other compassionate touches, but this one is uniquely ours. We've never even talked about this oddly intimate ritual but it's one of those things that make us who we are as a couple.

Now as I lay in bed with Jack I'm more and more conscious of his presence. I feel his breath on my face and run my hands over his skin. I dread the day that I won't be able to reach out and touch him, to know his warmth, to listen to his rhythmic breathing.

I feel fortunate that even though Jack is weak and obviously very sick, he hasn't lost his desire to be touched or to touch me. We still hold each other, he still reaches out for me, and I still get to renew my energy with his arms around me.

Coping

The salvo of seizures, hiccups, pain and never-ending test results make me feel like I'm suspended above a carpet of protruding shards of glass and know I'm going to lose my balance, plummet, and be pierced by pain. But my body won't feel the agony, only my heart. I'm afraid to move. Afraid to breath. If I just freeze in place the world might stop and Jack's symptoms won't progress. My heart won't be shattered into a million indistinguishable pieces that can never be mended.

So I try to ignore the dried blood caked in Jack's nostrils. I scrub years of our Mastiff's slobber-gobbers off the walls, not registering the rubber wheelchair marks that are the real reason I am washing the walls.

Sometimes, before Jack's seizure, when we made love in the morning and I was slated to work at home, I intentionally avoided showering so that Jack's smell stayed with me. I relived our intimacy through his smell long after he left the house. I'm petrified I'll be left with nothing that smells of Jack. So I take the stuffed bear that Jack's colleagues sent to him and make Jack use it as a pillow. He resists at first – he's not a stuffed bear person. But I tell him it's the best little head-sized pillow I've ever had. Sure enough, he starts using it. But it isn't capturing any smells.

A little help from our friends and family

When I try to manage communication and interactions with others, my brain engages in a tug of war with itself. Jack and I want to see friends and family, but we also don't want to see friends and family.

It's a distraction in time, energy and resources to get ready for visits. I pass most of the work off to Kiley and Conrad but I still have to play a part. I feel guilty putting more on them – it's not like this cancer isn't affecting their emotional health too.

It's because we have to put so much off on Kiley and Conrad that Jack has decided not to tell his brother, Jeff, that he has cancer until we get back to Baltimore. Jack wants to see Jeff but not while we are in Florida. He's hoping that when we return to Maryland Jeff will be able to come and visit us there.

Not only is planning for visits stressful, the actual visits tire Jack out and I fear seizures when Jack pushes himself too much. I don't know how to tell people it's time for them to leave. I'm sure they expect I will, but I can't.

And Jack has always been so sensitive to my needs that I'm not completely sure that he's being honest when we talk about visitors. I wonder if he says he wants to see people and do things just because he thinks that's what I want. So I have to explain to some people who want to visit that Jack's not strong enough and I don't even tell Jack I've turned our friends away. If I can't muster up the energy to entertain, I'm pretty sure he can't either.

In any case, it's definitely Jack who wants to see my parents.

Their 64th wedding anniversary is coming up and since we missed celebrating my father's birthday with him, Jack wants to get together with them. "Nancy, please call your dad and see if he can meet us at the Don Garlits Museum. I've always wanted to go there with him. Let's do it if he's able. See if John and Eileen can drive them up to Ocala."

Cane in his hand, cap on his head, and a smile on his face Jack greets my family. Like a kid running towards the county fair, he heads towards the museum.

I'm not sure it was a wonderful day for my mother though. Neither she nor I have any interest in the museum, so we go to a nearby coffee shop to play scrabble. Driving from the coffee shop back to the museum, I lose control.

My mother strongly believes in the power of prayer and talks about her perspective quite often. "I'm so glad God was good and has let us get together. He's answering our prayers and Jack is getting stronger."

Maybe it's because I didn't want her to be hopeful because I know Jack really isn't going to beat this cancer. Or maybe it's because I have never believed in praying for such concrete actions. Or maybe it's because all I could hear was – once again – no compliment to Jack. Whatever the reason, I explode. "Mom. It's *not* your prayers that are helping Jack. It's *Jack* who is helping Jack. His determination. His therapy. And it's the medicine. And the doctors. Please don't tell me anything about praying. I don't want to hear it."

My mother doesn't even look at me. Her head stays turned towards the road. She's silent. No retort. No contradiction. No "sermon" about how important it is to turn to God for support. She just remains quiet.

Immediately I know I have asked more of her than is fair to ask. I've disrespected her beliefs, raised my voice at her, and exposed my growing distance from my childhood religious practices. Gratefully my mother let me pass on this horrible breach of respect. No matter how upside-down my life is I have no right to yell at my mother.

When we reunite with the rest of the family, Conrad finds a fabulous Indian Restaurant by searching local eateries on his cell phone. What a digital era we live in. We talk and laugh together throughout dinner, after which, my parents, together with John and Eileen, head back south, and Jack, Conrad and I head home.

Packages keep coming from Jack's colleagues. I have only just written a note to Jing to thank her all for the wonderful gifts when ANOTHER package arrives. The boxes are so well timed. Jack loves the notes and the special treats. Besides taking care of Jack, Jing is taking care of me. How she knows I need slippers is beyond me – but I do.

Bess, back in Baltimore, organizes dinners to be delivered to our home in Gainesville. Our research team and a few people from UMBC pitch in, taking turns paying for meals we are able to order from local restaurants. "Doorstep Delivery" is someone's brainchild. All of us, especially Kiley and Conrad, feel thankful relief in being released from the demand to constantly shop and cook.

Our neighbors, Eric and Ann, have given me a baby monitor so that when Jack is sleeping I can move around the house and am able to hear him and help him when he wakes. Often when Jack takes naps I go outside and do yard work. I need to be in the sunshine. I need to do mindless work. I find great pleasure in pulling weeds out of our lawn and there are sure plenty there to keep me busy. Jack sleeps to heal while I wrench out the weeds by their roots, imagining my weeding as symbolically yanking the tumors out of Jack's body.

Jack wants to see my sister Carol and her husband, Bill. They come to be with us. To spend time with us. Carol makes arrangements and announces what we're doing when she's in town. They stay at a hotel, visit us at our home, and engaged in genuine conversation with us when we are together. I need no preplanning, there's no expense in terms of time or money, and there are no expectations for us to entertain them. When they offer to take us out to dinner, I decline the offer. I'm afraid to expose Jack to too many germs.

"Nancy, I want to go. I don't need to avoid a restaurant. The doctor said I can't swim, lift weights, or climb stairs. None of that's necessary to go out to eat."

Where I had initially thought these visits might have negative reverberations, I've been proven wrong. They are much needed.

John and Eileen have acted similarly. On one trip south, John and Eileen stop by our house in Maryland, set mousetraps, check in with the neighbors, and make sure our house is in complete order. Eileen even collects clothes I need and brings them to me. They have thought of details I have not considered.

When they are here visiting, our time is much like it is when Bill and Carol are here. John and Eileen take us out to dinner. We go to the same restaurant. We spend time laughing and talking, and cancer isn't the central focus of living.

I keep expecting Jack to "fall off the wagon" and have a beer with John but he doesn't. I'd have a drink again if I thought there was any way I could stop at just one, but since I know myself better than that, I continue to abstain.

Meeting friends and family is tiring but it helps Jack rebuild his stamina. Being with others in social environments is essential in our efforts to rebuild our emotional foundation that has been seriously abused over these past months. By mid-February Jack finally calls his former boss, Dr. Davis. Each year when we come back to Florida at Christmas time, we go out to dinner together. Our meeting this year was typical – dinner at Tim's Thai restaurant, catching up on our respective families, what Dr. Davis and his wife are enjoying doing during their retirement, and how Jack's research in the lab in Maryland has progressed. Talk about such routine matters never sounded so good.

Enough time has passed without a seizure and we've been out several times with others. Because of Carol and Bill, we're even taking a trip to Crystal River. Unselfishly, Carol convinces me to get a room at the Plantation Inn – it's not where we would normally stay. We usually stay with either Pat or Sue, or if we want our own accommodations, we stay at The Port. But Carol persuades me to go to the Plantation because she and Bill may be able to join us and it's a nicer place.

She's right. The resort is on a quiet part of the river, surrounded completely by water. It's exactly what Jack needs. I'm not sure if Carol ever intended to join us, but she and Bill have arranged and paid for the room for us. Jack and I enjoy three days making believe it's not the last time we'll visit Crystal River together.

When Gilly and Pandora, our friends since 1978, come from Belize to visit, I can't keep Jack home. We have breakfast, lunch and dinner together with our friends at our home and out at restaurants. We even make it to a play at the Hippodrome. I have been writing to Pandora since Terrible Tuesday. The emails help me express what I can't say, and because Pandora is and has been my friend for a long time I know she understands without making judgments. That's not to say my other friends and family don't also do that, but each relationship we have with the people we love should bring something special that's not shared with others.

Since Terrible Tuesday I've felt like I have fallen into a deep, dark well of despair. Since seeing Gilly and Pandora, I can change the image I've had of looking up and seeing nothing but darkness, to looking up to see Pandora smiling, hanging over the side of the well, looking down and calling out to me. "I'm here Nancy. I promise we can make it out of this mess." Standing behind Pandora is Gilly, with his hand on her leaning back, calling to Jack to come up and have a laugh with him.

To see Jack two weeks ago and then to see him now is amazing. He couldn't talk, walk, or use his right hand at all. Now he is talking, walking and has only to strengthen his hand and fine-tune his motor skills. Even the tremors are better every day. We think they might settle on their own too. He's down from 45 mg to 30 mg of morphine twice a day. And he's eating well.

Dr. Engle

Dr. Engle treats Jack as a colleague in research. Dr. Hyland must have known this would be the case when he steered Jack to Dr. Engle for outpatient care.

Jack likes the straightforward, scientific, fact-based approach Dr. Engle uses when he reports Jack's progress. "The lymph node is shrinking. The pain is expected and related to the flare of the disease. The tumor in the lung is more than fifty percent decreased."

This is all good news. I like hearing it too. Unfortunately, he doesn't stop there.

"The cyst on the kidney has stayed the same. There are small, slow-growing renal tumors that we are not pursuing now. At the end of your treatment if there's still the one area of question on the kidney we will pursue it then. We will also monitor the tumor on the liver."

What? The kidney and liver are *involved?* Jack just listens. I have no idea what to say or how to say it so I just write everything down. I vaguely remember Dr. Hyland commenting something about cysts but no one followed up on that and I never asked for more information. My hands start to shake and it's hard to concentrate. I just keep writing because Dr. Engle doesn't stop.

Dr. Engle's voice is steady. He keeps his gaze focused on Jack. He's really very professional. "Your strength is good. You are feeling well, that's part of the decision-making process for continued treatment. We will plan another infusion."

Jack's face doesn't change. I bet this is what he looks like in his own lab – listen, think, plan, act.

"Your white counts are a little low so we may delay your next treatment. We can give you shots to raise your count artificially but that doesn't protect the patient and I tend not to use them."

I experience the same yoyo feelings I had before when we got mixed messages from different sources:

Good news – the tumor in your lung is in a good location for surgery.

Bad news – oops, stage four, no surgery option.
Good news – this drug might help your hiccups.
Bad news – it's psychotropic and doesn't even work once tried.
Good news – the tumors are shrinking.
Bad news – your kidney and liver have problems.
Good news – we will continue treatment.
Bad news – there will be a delay…

Jack's cognitive confusion is better all the time but there are two areas that are just too stubborn. One is that he still has a hard time comprehending what he reads. He won't let me read to him and he won't listen to our audio book yet.

The other is in understanding some explanations. He has a hard time when I pose situations that require a choice. He can't follow more abstract comments that require contextualization. For example, as we drove past an Indian restaurant I said to him, "If that restaurant we went to in Ocala was here in Gainesville, we would have returned to it already." The comment is situational but Jack should have known what I meant. It took me three times of saying it and explaining it before he understood. When he finally "got it" he acted like I left out most of the information in the earlier statements, even though I had repeated myself almost verbatim.

Jack's blood counts are not very strong. His third chemo, scheduled for February 23, has to be postponed.

Business NOT as usual

So many times I look at Jack and see how strong he has become and how much he's fighting back that I'm sure the doctors are wrong and he is going to live much longer than six months. Jack and I listened to the statistics and we know that Jack's chances are not good, but we don't talk about him succumbing to the cancer.

Physical and occupational therapy, as well as Jack's determination to recover his strength, fine motor skills, and mobility have made a difference. He has fought back from a month in a wheel chair with little use of his right side. He needs to keep working to build strength, stamina, fine motor dexterity, and endurance, but Matt, his home-care physical therapist, basically fired Jack because he has reached a point where he needs more aggressive therapy. We're shifting from home care to a PT center.

Even without the explicit language of death, the emotional twists are constant. One hour Jack is talking and laughing and the next hour he's tired and I can see him struggling not to show he's feeling poorly. I know how important it is for me to stay hopeful and positive, and not discuss the doctors' prediction that only a few months of life is a possibility. Jack and I are researchers –we know what outliers are, and we want Jack to be one. I smile when Jack says, "We're in this for the long haul."

But deep in my heart I know it's not likely. I keep smiling. I keep hoping. I keep making sure I do as much for Jack's healing as I can. But I don't pray. I'm leaving that to my mother.

CHAPTER 14

Return To Maryland

March 1 – March 13

In one of the books my sister Carol got for us to read, *Cutting for Stone* written by Abraham Verghese, I find a line that makes me stop reading and think. "There is a point when grief exceeds the human capacity to emote, and as a result one is strangely composed." I hope Jack and Conrad see me as *composed*, but inside I'm anything but. We have decided it's time to get back to Maryland.

I'm doing the best I can and will continue to do so, but I'm scared out of my mind almost all the time. I make a note:

Fear

Fear storms in and anchors herself in my life. She is a bully, relentlessly beating me down. Her hallow eyes bore into me. Each time I find strength enough to look for *Hope*, *Fear* clamps her fist around my heart and squeezes. Strength motivates her. *Fear* lurks in the shadows casting darkness into the future. She devours everything that is good. She battles *Confidence* and wins every encounter. Power emanates from her every move causing all to bow to her authority.

Jack is my soul mate, my best friend, half my brain and all my memory. The thought of losing him is terrifying. If the doctors are right, we have a very limited number of days. Jack wants to plan our trip back to Maryland. He wants to get back to work.

Jack's blood counts pass and his third chemo infusion starts our month. We need to schedule our travel around Jack's chemo so that we'll have time to settle in, get new doctors, and have a good direction for care. Jack has made all the progress he can with the therapists here. He's ready to head north.

Dr. Engle is right about Hospice, it's been good to have their support. Before leaving, *Haven Hospice* helps me find contacts for Hospice in Maryland. Unlike here in Alachua County, there are many options in Baltimore County and we have to make a choice. I want to complete the arrangements before we get back to Maryland so that I don't lose this kind of help. That means choosing care before we've met key personnel or seen the facilities. But we must have help upon our arrival in Maryland, so we do as much research as possible and make a choice. Jack will enroll in Gilchrist Hospice as soon as we get back.

We also pick up Jack's records, films and scans from Shands radiology. We need to walk into Jack's new oncology office with everything in hand so that Jack's care is continuous.

Over the past few weeks I've been working together with Jack's boss, Alan, and it's all set – Jack will see a physician who he has done research with in the past. The doctor, Caleb Bergoff, is one of the best lung cancer oncologists at UMMC where Jack will seek treatment.

Jack's primary goal is to get back to work. He's not able to consider returning full time at this point, but he wants to see what he can do once we return. He's anxious to see his colleagues. Everyone from his lab has been so supportive, sending cards, emails and care packages.

Alan has also agreed to let Jack work however much he can – even if it's a few hours a day, a few days a week to start. We'll need to fit work in around doctor appointments and his fourth chemo, which is scheduled for March 22. At this point Jack is leaning towards transferring all his medical oncology to UMMC, but he wants to return in early April to Shands if he can for the MRI to follow up with his brain scan.

It's unusual for me to be the one to pack the car. This has always been Jack's job. I love my little car – it has a huge trunk and I know I can manage the packing.

"You're never going to fit all your shit in the car Nancy." Jack has no confidence in me.

Conrad chuckles. "Do you want help Mom? I think Dad's right – you're going to have to leave some of your things here."

"Well if you hadn't picked a hundred grapefruit when we were in Crystal River you would be able to fit my clothes." Jack continues to express his doubt.

Determined to prove Jack wrong, I spend two days packing the car. I use small bags for most of our belongings so that I can fill every nook and cranny in the trunk. I pack the large duffle bag that Jack teasingly calls the "body bag" full so it's firm. I situate it on the back seat. Juno will have to share the seat, but she's such a compliant dog. I'm sure she'll have no trouble.

We're all packed. Just before we head to the car, we are both in the bedroom but my back is to Jack.

"Nancy," Jack's voice sounds solemn.

I turn and see Jack holding his boat keys, which I've never been privy to because it's *Jack's* boat. "Just in case," he says as he drops the keys in the drawer of the bureau. Jack lowers his eyes and I turn away from him so he doesn't see my tears.

Normally we spend one night on the road between Florida and Maryland but for this trip we've planned two nights and three days travel. We know the hotels where we can stop with Juno and we're hoping that if all goes well, we can drive from Gainesville to Florence, South Carolina to Rocky Mount, North Carolina, and then on the third day, arrive in Baltimore.

As we drive north on March 5, the geographic changes seem to match my mood. We are leaving behind blue skies, fresh air and warm breezes. The farther north we drive, the cloudier the skies. We stop at every rest area and walk around. Slowly. Jack isn't well, but he's managing to keep his spirits high. We listen to the audio book we started on our way down, Michael Crichton's *Micro*, but only in short bursts – not for chapters at a time like we did back in December.

The first night we make it as planned – Florence, South Carolina. I've packed dinner so that we don't have to go out to a restaurant, and Jack is so tired that after we eat, Jack walks Juno while I clean up the dinner mess, then we watch TV for just an hour and call it a night.

The second day of driving is much like the first. The traffic isn't bad, the book keeps us somewhat engaged, and we stop at all the rest areas to take short walks. Jack needs the walks but so does Juno. This is her second day riding in the back seat. She's used to more space but since we traded in the SUV, the back seat is all she gets.

Jack doesn't want to stop for the night at our usual place in Rocky Mount, things are going well and he wants to try to get a little farther north. He finds a Marriot in Emporia, Virginia in our *AAA Tour Book* and calls to make sure they have a room and will accept Juno. So we keep driving another sixty miles. By the time we get to the Marriott, Jack is tired, but otherwise all seems okay.

When we awake for our third day of travel, Jack is sick. He's not getting out of bed. I quickly walk Juno and rush back to the room to make sure Jack is okay. He's sound asleep. I hurry to the lobby to get breakfast. Jack is still asleep. I take a chance once more and with great urgency speak to the front desk manager to make sure the room is available one more night. It is.

I read while Jack sleeps. The hotel is nice enough, but it's not as nice as the one in Rocky Mount. I question myself – maybe I should not have let Jack push us this far. It's so damn hard to know what to do. Mistakes are not little anymore. A small error in judgment can cause a maelstrom of problems.

Jack wakes about noon. We take Juno for a walk and he has a sandwich.

"Let's drive into town to see what this place is like," he suggests.

I'm shocked. We traveled for Conrad's sports events for two decades and Jack never wanted to look around little towns.

We get flyers from the hotel lobby, take our map and the *AAA Tour Book*, and head out for a drive. After about an hour of "looking around" I'm getting sick of trying to figure out why Jack has all-of-a sudden become a small-town sightseer when he shifts back to his more normal self. "Well this is an interesting enough little place. I've seen enough. Have you?"

"Yes and I'm really surprised you wanted to see any of it. What's up with that?" I smile as he looks at me. He knows he's busted.

"I just don't want to just sit in the hotel all day and I don't feel well enough to try to get to Maryland. This let me get back in the car to see if I could handle it and gave us something to look at. You don't mind, do you?"

"Of course I don't mind. I like looking at old churches. The courthouse was interesting and I liked learning a bit about this city's commerce."

All I said to Jack is true but in my mind I'm worried about the next and last leg of the trip. I've decided not to try to go through DC. Jack hates DC and I don't need anything irritating him. Also, if we drive up 301 I'll be able to stop at any of the little towns along the route.

In theory it's a good idea. But once behind the wheel I wonder if I've made another mistake. It's a longer drive. I'm anxious. I want to be home. Even though I think I have good reason to speed, the police don't.

I'm driving 70 in a 55 zone when police sirens sound behind me.

Juno rocks the car barking and lunging at the window I've cracked to be able to hear the policeman. I ask him if I can please step out of the car to speak to him. Granted permission, I lean against the car, hand him my license and registration, and feel all emotion drain from my body. "I wish I could explain why I was speeding, but I can't. I just don't have the strength."

The cop stays as stoic as any policeman with whom I have ever interacted. He just looks at me, and without words, accepts the documents I hand to him.

Tears roll down my cheeks. I wait as he walks back to his car to do what I know he's going to do. When he returns I just take the ticket, get back in the car and drive away.

We make it back to Baltimore before dark. That's all I was hoping for. I take time to unload the car, one bag at a time. Jack gets situated in the house and gratefully, I realize I have a few dinners in the freezer – I'm not going to have to cook.

I've never known how much work it is to make these trips. My leg muscles hurt from carrying so much weight up the stairs. I realize the return to Maryland signals yet another change in our normal routines – I've become the manual laborer of the household. Jack can't do it and Conrad's in Florida.

Tonight I lay my head on my pillow in my own home. We made it. With Juno on her bed on one side of me and Jack lying in the bed on the other side, I am comforted by the loud sounds of stereo snoring.

In like a lion

So far, March is living up to its reputation. Sunday, March 11, just three days after Jack and I get back to Maryland, John drives down for an afternoon and then turns right back around to go back to Poughkeepsie. He does it so that he can show himself and us that it's possible to zip down at a moment's notice if we need help.

Monday Jack and I drive to the other side of Baltimore so Jack can meet with Steve. We give Steve a copy of Jack's medical files. Steve doesn't practice out of UMMC but Jack can still see him as an outpatient if he needs to. We also drop a complete file of all Jack's records from Shands off at the oncologist's office at UMMC who will manage Jack's care.

Tuesday the Gilchrist Hospice social worker comes to our house. Jack enrolls in the program, and I silently thank Dr. Engle for helping us accept help from Hospice.

CHAPTER 15

The Strength To Face Each Moment

I often wonder if Jack's sheer determination to go back to work through all of his pain and struggle is somehow related to his determination to be a happy person in spite of some of the trials he faced in his relationship with his mother, Jerry.

Over the years, no matter what, Jack did not speak ill of his mother. After she presented us with the bill for his upbringing, he not only made regular payments to her but he also continued to interact with her. She visited us as often as we could manage, usually twice a year and almost always during the Thanksgiving/Christmas holidays, coming from her home in St. Petersburg to Gainesville, usually by bus, and staying with Jack and me at our home.

Because of her history of drinking, Jack was always on guard to make sure that she didn't have alcohol in our home, but it was never a problem. She continued to smoke cigarettes, but she respected our wishes and smoked only outside our house.

What she never seemed able to do was to respect Jack. She criticized him for what seemed like every accomplishment he managed. Our apartment was too small and the air conditioner didn't keep it very cool, his new car was too expensive, the dinners I cooked were not appetizing, our first home needed too much work and wasn't on the right side of town. "Jack, don't you remember what your father used to say – 'Location, location, location.'" Jack kept quiet and never argued with his mother. But he finally hit his limit.

Conrad was in first grade and Jerry had come up to Gainesville to spend three days with us for a Christmas visit. Her bus arrived in the late afternoon. I picked her up, brought her to our home, and helped her settle in. About four o'clock Jack called me from his lab and asked me if he could work late because he needed more time to get emotionally ready for his mother's visit.

From the time I hung up the phone, assuring Jack I was fine and that he could come home when he was ready, until seven o'clock when I heard his car pull into our driveway, I found myself defending every decision Jack and I had made in recent years. Why was Conrad in Catholic school – could we afford the tuition? When was I going to get a professional job so that I could contribute to the family income? Why didn't Jack apply for other jobs so that he could earn a higher salary? The questions were not part of a conversation. They were part of an assault.

When Jack walked in the door, I looked him in the eyes, said, "It's your turn. I'm going to Becky's. I'll be back later. I'm sorry Jack. I tried."

At nine o'clock I walked through our back door into the family room. Jack was watching TV. Gently I asked, "Where's your mother?"

"She's in her room. She's changed her bus tickets. You'll take her to the bus station the first thing tomorrow morning. We'll talk about this after I get home from work tomorrow, okay?"

How odd, I thought. This was really nothing like Jack. But I honored his wishes, and waited a day to find out that, while I was having a glass of ice tea with my friend, Jerry had started asking Jack the same questions she had posed to me all over again. And she didn't stop there. When she said, "Your son is spoiled, he doesn't need that bicycle, he has too many toys, he has too many things," Jack happened to be walking through the living room and saw the look on Conrad's face and turned back to face his mother and told her to stop. He told me he said, "You ruined my childhood. You will not do that to my son. Nancy will take you to the bus station in the morning. You are not welcome in my home anymore."

The strength it took for Jack to be Jerry's son might have provided the foundation he needed to fight his way back from four seizures, hand paralysis, distorted speech and immobilizing hip pain. One never knows why we are who we are, but surely Jack's way of turning away from conflict has its roots somewhere. So does his smile.

On March 14, he is ready and able to work. Jack is back in his lab.

CHAPTER 16

New Doctor, New Approach

March 19

The yoyo ride continues. There's little that will carry over from Jack's care in Florida besides the general diagnosis that he has stage four lung cancer, but even that's something this new doc, Caleb Bergoff, wants to double check on his own.

Our new way of looking at life is that we're working for "disease stability" with "progression free survival" as the goal. Our first impression is that Dr. Bergoff may be more aggressive in his approach than Dr. Engle. He refuses to sign the necessary papers for Jack to be in Hospice care, saying, "You don't need Hospice yet. You have a good year or two before that."

When Jack and I hear these words we both break out into smiles that are full of energy. We instantly lock eyes with each other and Jack's voice is chipper when he says, "Well that's a nice change from what we heard in Florida."

Dr. Bergoff has signed the necessary forms for Jack to continue working "as tolerated." This gives Jack the ability to work when he can and not work when he can't. We don't know what working part time means in terms of Jack's Social Security Disability benefits, but I'll see what I can find out to make sure we're not left in a lurch should "progression" occur – which would mean the cancer is growing again.

Jack's performance status is Level One – that's really good. His cancer is not "progression free" at this point, and Dr. Bergoff won't discuss Jack's exact prognosis until he has his own testing complete. None of the doctors we've interacted with are comfortable predicting life expectancy, but Bergoff said that Jack's original prognosis of three to six months doesn't seem right. In eight days, it will have been three months since Jack's first seizure.

Bergoff is testing for more mutations and other types of disease markers that have just become known in the field (actually in the last six weeks). Jack's fourth chemo is delayed by four days because the office couldn't get the insurance information in place soon enough to keep to the original date. Bergoff is following the same chemical routine that Engle used, though I get the sense that Bergoff may have decided on a different chemical composition or course of treatment should he have been the first to make the decisions.

There are other differences too. Dr. Engle supports maintenance chemotherapy after the initial treatment phase, Bergoff does not. Bergoff prefers to give his patients a "drug holiday" – he has followed the research and says that there's not an extended life expectancy from maintenance chemotherapy, as long as the patient is closely monitored when on his drug vacation. Regular checks (six to eight weeks), scans, and blood tests are a must while on vacation.

Unlike Engle, Bergoff will use the "shot" (I'm not sure what the med is called) to elevate Jack's white blood cell count should it be needed for Monday's chemotherapy. That was something Engle did not like using, he preferred Jack wait until his body restored the white blood cell count on its own. Given this approach, Jack is most likely to have the treatments on time. Like Engle, Bergoff will check after the fourth chemo cycle to make sure Jack's tumor is responding and still shrinking before he agrees to cycles five and six. There's great discussion/concern about the cumulative, toxic effects of the treatment. They call this the "clinical benefit ratio," and will only make decisions as the treatment is administered to make sure Jack isn't losing feeling in his hands and feet and other functions that would greatly reduce his quality of life. Bergoff also wants Jack off Dilantin – something the Florida neurologists used as their primary anti-seizure drug.

Another difference between the two doctors is dealing with the brain metastases (mets). In Florida, the neurosurgeons who did Jack's radio surgery were strict about a three-month follow up and immediate treatment should more brain mets develop. Bergoff's approach is to complete the chemotherapy and then conduct whole brain radiation. The Florida doctors discouraged whole brain radiation because of the possible side effects (memory loss or worse). Jack had seizures partially because of the treatment and partially because of the brain mets. The physicians will present the treatment options to Jack, but in the end, Jack will be the one to say which treatment he will request, although at present he's undecided on whether he should choose the whole brain radiation or the stereotactic radiation. We'll be referred to radiation oncologists who will go over this with us more before we have to make a decision – but in the meantime, I suppose we'll miss the three-month MRI that the Florida doctors felt was very important.

Neither Jack nor I are comfortable missing the three-month follow up MRI. Brain mets cause seizures and seizures scare the hell out of both of us. But we have learned that no amount of insistence and no number of questions will advance the rate at which Jack will receive tests and treatments. So we deal with our disappointment in silence.

There's agreement on a few other issues:

1. Jack will not get the drugs to strengthen his bones. The risk for necrosis of the jaw is too great because of Jack's dental bone graft (done in December before we left Maryland).

2.　Jack still should not drive. There's been no discussion whether or not driving will ever be an option for Jack. I believe we need to have further discussion with the neurologist about this issue. In Florida we were under the impression we just had to wait to be seizure free for six months but here in Maryland there was no discussion about that – just a flat "No."

3.　Jack needs plenty of rest, to continue to avoid alcohol, and to maintain a healthy diet. A safe exercise routine would greatly improve his quality of life.

4.　While undergoing chemotherapy Jack's temperature needs to be monitored – anything over 100°F warrants a direct trip to the doctor's office or ER if after hours.

5.　A week to a week and a half after chemo is the period of time Jack has to be extra careful about germs – he's most immuno-compromised at that time because his white blood cells are destroyed by the treatment.

There was a concern about renal cell carcinoma in Jack's records from Florida which was also expressed by Dr. Engle at our last visit. I finally understand this complication. The scans in Florida all indicate that Jack's renal cysts are simple – not malignant. They'll be monitored closely, just like the rest of Jack's body. Should they change, the course of treatment would most likely be surgery but Jack would be referred to a different oncologist should the need develop.

Dr. Bergoff is personable and the people in his practice are pleasant and seem competent, but it's very different being in Baltimore City. At this point I don't feel switching to UMMC will negatively compromise Jack's care. It's emotionally taxing and it's hard to deal with the difference of opinions (especially when it comes to the brain mets) but I don't think we can know who is right and who isn't – or even if there's a "not right" approach. We do have to believe that someone is closest to the *truth*, but we don't feel that going back and forth between Maryland and Florida care will buy us much.

Worry

I don't know if this is normal or not but I worry a great deal about Jack dying. I worry that my worrying is counter-productive and feeds negative energy, but I can't stop what pops into my mind. One of my biggest fears is that I won't remember my life with Jack because he's my memory. He reminds me of experiences we've shared that I just don't seem to be able to recall myself.

CHAPTER 17

Holding On

March 15 – April 22

You realize what is really important in your life when you are held hostage over a long period of time. Cancer is holding me hostage. Jack's illness, his treatment and care, and the unlikelihood of him recovering from this disease is changing how I see the world.

Every morning that I wake up and Jack is coherent, able to smile, get out of bed, and pet Juno is a gift. It's been this way all our lives but the gift is now a conscious one that sparkles, stands out and is very much what I long for. Time. That is what has become most precious to me.

Jack's gift is normalcy. When he was first diagnosed, I offhandedly, but with a great deal of caution, had asked him whether or not he wanted to make a bucket list.

"Nancy, I don't have a bucket list. I have lived a good life. I've done what I wanted to do, seen what I wanted to see." He paused long enough for me to realize that he is really a very contented man. His years of living a life of routine, of being a steady, thoughtful person have served him very well. He is and has been a pleasant person. Someone who others enjoy being around because of his level-headed ways. "No," he continued, "I don't have a list of things I want to do, but I might like to make a list of all the things I want to eat before I die."

With this denial, I even more cautiously observe him. My goal is to give Jack what he wants, which is to give as little attention to his cancer as possible. He wants to wake up, S-S-and S as he as always called it ("shit shower and shave") and get on with his day. He wants me to drive him to work using the same route he used. He wants me to park his car in the same lot where he has always parked. He wants to take the same shuttle. He wants to play the same games he always played on his colleagues – sneaking up on Christie early in the morning and turning off the lab lights, putting lab supplies up on the top shelf, too high for Li to reach, and taping various cartoons on people's doors so they start their days with a smile.

At home he wants to do the grocery shopping, take out the garbage, set the coffee, and care for Juno and Hei Mei. But he can't do it all. His stamina expires. His concentration wanes.

I can't pick up the slack. I'm tired. When fatigue overtakes me, I call Conrad and ask him to make a trip north.

Side effects

One of the side effects of Jack's chemo is neuropathy. First Jack's feet and ankles, then his hands have become numb and tingly. Every night while we watch our movie, I strip off his shoes and socks and rub his feet and legs to help circulate the blood and stimulate his nerve endings so that he'll get his normal feeling back. It often hurts a little when I first start rubbing him, but with time it feels better. Jack feels progress. He's getting more feeling in his feet so he welcomes my foot massages.

Now the neuropathy is starting to hit Jack's hands. He's becoming more concerned, but rather than give in to the symptom, he's going to our acupuncturist. I wonder why none of Jack's oncologists, either at Shands or UMMC, have told Jack to do this, because the acupuncture really does help.

Acupuncture doesn't help the freaking hiccups though. The longest we seem to be able to control them has been one week. Jack enjoyed one glorious week of no jerking and no spasms. He didn't have to induce vomiting and could keep all the calories he ingested. But they are back. When the hiccups finally stopped I felt like we were defying the odds, but now that they are back my feelings of defeat are worse than ever. I hate this disease. I don't want Jack losing more and more physical functioning of his body and I don't want him in pain. And I worry about myself. How am I going to manage if Jack dies and I am left alone?

Like Hemingway who, in *Green Hills of Africa*, confessed to lying awake at night missing Africa before he had even left the country, I miss Jack before he has even died. I imagine myself alone in our bed, wondering what it will be like to wake up in the morning and have no Jack here to say "Good Morning Honey" to. I doubt I will be able to manage without him.

Intimacy

When Jack and I met, I had a waterbed. I've never been willing to give it up, but I didn't insist on having one in both our homes. Returning to Maryland has the special treat of returning to our bed where we are both much more comfortable. The bed is heated, and for the first time in our lives, Jack needs more heat than I. Our bed is our haven.

The softness of the mattress brings us closer together and more intimate than when we lie next to each other in any other bed. Our years of sexual pleasure are more alive, and Jack has recovered enough to surprise me in the middle of the night, exploring my body once again, arousing me, gently holding me, and making the softest, most meaningful love that we have ever shared.

Siblings

Being a wife and caregiver has been my life for months. I know it's affected me in many ways. It has changed my thinking, my purpose, my energy, my sleeping. My everything.

Even being a sister. In the past, when I've identified my roles and relationships I've always listed wife, mother, daughter, sister. I never thought of the role of "sister" multiplied by four, I was just a sister.

Unexpected feelings and energy concerning my siblings emerge every day. It's so odd to me that each of my ties with my brothers and sisters is so distinctive. And they are constantly changing.

Jeanne, who has always taken a sort-of-mother role in my life, continues in that same way. She wants to make sure that I'm not denying the inevitable. She points out that Jack's cancer is terminal. She tells me it's important to start figuring out my financial status now, and that waiting isn't an option. She and Andre visit us again and we go out to dinner, to a play at the theater in Olney, and we play dominoes. I pretend to be okay. One night after Andre and Jack go to bed, I sit up with Jeanne and do as she advises and review my financial challenges. But as soon as she and Andre leave to go back to New York I put the papers on the bottom of the work piles in my study where I won't see them again unless I dig all the way to China.

Chuck, who has always been the most distant of all my siblings, also remains the same. He sends heart-felt emails and responds to communications I send. But he's in the shadows, where he has placed himself throughout most of my life. Jack and Chuck have always gotten along when they are together, but in all these years Chuck has only come to visit us one time and that was when his children were young. We have never gone together to Maine to visit Chuck, though I have gone there without Jack more than once. When Conrad was in elementary school Jack and I had a litter of pups. They were beautiful yellow Labradors, healthy, with a great lineage. Eventually we gave Abel to Chuck.

John and Carol have been playing such active roles in my life that I know I would not be as strong as I am without them. But even their roles are entirely dissimilar.

John and his wife Eileen have brought me so much comfort I don't think I can even find the words to explain my feelings. The role they have in my life isn't one I knew could exist before Terrible Tuesday. I feel compassion, understanding, and respect.

Neither John nor Eileen has uttered a single word that has upset me. They don't ask questions that are too hard to think about – let alone answer. They never say, "What can we do for you?" Instead, they intuitively know what Jack and I need.

John is the closest of my siblings to us geographically, but that closeness matters only if he's demonstrated his willingness to travel the distance, which he's done. He tells me when he's not going to be home for any length of time so that if I need him, I won't panic if I can't reach him by phone.

In mid-April we meet at Antietam Battle Field in Sharpsburg and spend the day walking around the fields, talking and laughing all the time. I could not make this trip alone with Jack, but it's a lot of fun to be able to go with John and Eileen. When Jack gets completely disoriented and insists we turn away from the center of town and I can't convince him we aren't going to make it to the restaurant driving in this direction, I pull off the road and let John help Jack understand we need to turn around. Once at the pub, we spend the evening enjoying the crazy atmosphere, good food, and yelling young people all around us. These days are like pockets of calm in the midst of turbulent seas.

Like John and Eileen, Carol has made regular visits both with and without her husband Bill. While I seek comfort in John's time with us, I sap strength out of my relationship with Carol. Carol's relationship with Jack has been a good one. It's a real friendship, one that is special to Carol and to Jack. Carol has always spent time with us. In fact, she is my only sibling who attended Jack's and my wedding. When I see her kindness and affection towards Jack I know her feelings are true and honest.

When she comes to visit it's the most natural time I feel. We do normal things together like we've always done – plant spring flowers, clear out my over-stuffed closet, take the dog for a walk, and now, drop Jack off at work and even visit with his colleagues because Jack wants Carol to see his lab and insists that she meet his lab wife, Jing. Introducing Carol to his peers and touring her around his lab is something Jack would only do if he truly loves and honors Carol.

She comes to visit often enough that she knows I'm barely holding on. "Nancy, you've lost yourself. You don't care about work, you don't care about your friends, and you don't care about much of anything besides making it through the day. But you need to care. Yes, though a car could hit you tomorrow and you might die, the odds are much greater that you are going to have to learn to live your life without Jack physically at your side. To do that, you need to make sure you have interests that get you out of your skin, out of your house, and out of your growing depression."

Her words force me to try and push away the paralysis of fear that has gripped me. She's the only person who can (and does) snap me into thinking about day-to-day living. I invite Bess for lunch. Jack and I go to Morna and Len's kids' birthday party. We go to Meghan's for dinner. I try to pick up my academic work and write. I try but I fail.

She knows it too. But still she texts me daily, emails more often, and when she tells me, "I am here for you both whenever you need me," I know she means exactly what she says.

Jack has spoken to his brother on the phone on a couple of occasions. He has told Jeff that he has cancer, that it's stage four, and describes the various organs that have been affected. He's talked about the treatments he's received and is still receiving. I know Jack wants Jeff to come visit, but he won't ask him to make the trip. Jack has not talked to him about longevity, and I don't know if Jeff understands the severity of Jack's disease. One thing I'm sure of, this is not something I'll interfere in. Jack and I have always talked to each other about our siblings, about our relationships with them, and how we might or might not handle a specific situation. But he has never disrespected the decisions I have made concerning the Rankies and I have never disrespected those he has made concerning the Sheltons.

Every aspect of living changes

In my previous life, every Saturday morning Jack would fill our vehicles with gas. When he first started this practice I argued with him. "Jack, I don't drive that much. I don't need gas every week."

"I know, Nancy. But this way we keep the tank full just in case you get one of your wild hairs and want to drive up to Pennsylvania and visit Xenia or something. And besides that, we keep our budget more balanced from week to week. Unless, of course, you make one of your spur-of-the-moment trips."

Now, in this new life, I'm the only driver and I can't seem to get into a routine that includes stopping at a gas station on a regular basis. It scares me because I certainly would not be able to stop for gas on the way to the ER should the need arise. For the first few weeks we were here in Maryland I was able to just trade off the two vehicles, driving one for a week and then changing to drive the other.

Then one day about three weeks after we returned from Florida, I slid into the driver's seat at 7:35 AM and started the SUV with purpose. Jack had an appointment at UMMC at 8 AM. We barely had enough time and Jack was moving slower and slower. There would be no more rushing from car to building. The gas tank registered less than a quarter of a tank. I broke out in a sweat and decided right then and there that one of the vehicles had to go.

That day I called Conrad. "Please fly up to Baltimore as soon as possible. I need you to get a one-way ticket. I want you to take the Benz back to Florida with you, please. Can you do that?"

"Of course I will, Mom. But why?"

"I just can't manage to keep both cars up. I need to feel like I'm in control and I can't feel that way if I'm worried about which vehicle has gas or which one should be parked in the driveway first."

"Is Dad going to be okay with me taking his new car? You know how proud of it he is."

"Dad will understand. I can't keep both and if we need to rush Dad to the hospital we can't do it in the Benz."

With just one car the stress is reduced as far as not having to keep up with two gas tanks, but buying gas requires overcoming feelings of desperation. Though I want to believe Jack's brain mets are shrinking and there are no new ones, he's too confused for me to keep lying to myself. He insists on pumping the gas and since we're always together, I can't circumvent his wishes by just going to the gas station myself. When Jack tries to do very normal things like pump gas, he can't. He's put the wrong grade of gas in the tank, he's forgotten to get receipts, he's spilled gas on himself and the car. You name it – however one can mess up pumping gas Jack has done it.

I'm tired all the time. Sleeping at night is nearly impossible. If I'm not freaking out that Jack's hand is twitching, which I know is another brain mets symptom, then the darn dog keeps me awake. Juno, a 145-pound Mastiff, snores as loud as any human I have ever heard. I'm afraid she'll wake Jack with her snoring or her pacing.

I try to nap when Jack naps, but I rarely can. So I sip tea and try to read. I want to become a character in my book. Repeatedly I have read about people in distress who are "waiting to wake up and find this is all a bad dream" only to rouse and find everything is the same. With Jack's cancer, I too wonder when I am going to awaken from the nightmare Jack and I are living. I might be in a semi-conscious daze, sleeping, or even wide-awake and aware, or watching Jack sleep, or waiting for him to come back from one test or another, when I ask myself what reality is. Am I really living this nightmare or can the world change back to my old normal life? But I never "wake up" to things even being the same, let alone waking up to something better.

For us, things are perpetually getting worse. Jack's disease is attacking him so fast, so hard. Jack knows this too and every time he is knocked back he just musters the strength to keep fighting. When other people comment on his "latest" diagnosis, he just says, "And the hits just keep on coming." At first I could smile with him but eventually I've come to realize I'll never again know a day anything like the days we shared before Terrible Tuesday.

Jack is relying on morphine now on a regular basis. It's become part of his daily medication. Just like the Keppra, I know this is a med he will take for the rest of his life. But he gets up every day, dresses, has breakfast, and I drive him to work. I cannot leave him there because of the threat of seizures, or even collapse. So we park, walk to his building, and then Jack goes to the elevator and up to his lab while I settle in the lobby for the duration. I spend the time trying to read academic literature in order to get my head back into my work and I write as much as I can to contribute to the book Bess and I are editing. It's almost impossible for me to focus, but I do my best.

When is a cold not a cold? When it's life threatening. Then a cold is more than a cold. It's death. I cover my mouth with three layers of tissues when I cough. I wash my hands every time I need to touch something. I have Clorox wipes on every floor and use them constantly to try to sterilize the house. The doctors tell me it's counter-productive to worry because I was infectious before I had symptoms. But I can't help it. I know Jack's body probably can't fight off a simple common cold.

Maybe it's because I'm sick I finally find the courage to tell Jack that I don't think it's fair that he's giving everything good he has to his job and not me. I ask him if we can take a vacation together. Something more than a day trip to Sharpsburg.

"Nancy I don't want to spend the money we would need to spend on traveling. I don't like traveling like you like it. And I don't want to be too far away from my doctors."

I completely understand these points. Since I think Jack is listening I try sharing another of my concerns. "I think it's counter-productive to set an early alarm for you to go to work. You need your rest and you can go in to the lab later in the morning and still contribute."

"Okay, I'll set the alarm for 6:30 instead of 6:00."

"Big whoop. Why not get up at eight, get to work at nine, come home at one?"

"No. It's unfair to work just those few hours and spend lunch on the job."

I swear he's driving me crazy with his concern about fairness and this self-perceived proper way to behave. But in spite of my frustration, I can say we are setting new records in our marriage. We haven't argued at all since Terrible Tuesday, and we are not going to either. So we are making constant progress... even if it's not exactly the progress I would like to see.

Tonight when I am in bed next to Jack, he's sound asleep and his breathing sounds deep and healthy. He turns his body towards me, lying on his side, which is unusual. I turn to my side, facing him, and feel the warmth of his breath. I time my own breathing so that I inhale the warm air he exhales.

I stay like this for several minutes. The cadence of Jack's breathing together with the oddness of my thoughts is comforting. I know it's irrational, but I suppose that if we can keep breathing in rhythm like this long enough that when Jack dies I'll always have his breath in me to sustain his presence in my life.

CHAPTER 18

UMMC Is No Shands

April 23 – May 26

Keeping up with Jack's care is much more like it was the first months dealing with this cancer in Gainesville. But it's much more complicated here.

First, I can't call the ambulance if Jack needs to go to the ER. Baltimore and Baltimore County first responder policy is to transport the patient to the geographically closest hospital. St. Agnes Hospital ER is the closest to our home, but all of Jack's doctors are coordinated out of UMMC, so I have to get him to the UMMC ER on my own.

I've enlisted a neighbor's help, William. He's a retired vet and quite strong, a genuinely nice man. When I need him I just call and he comes to drive us directly to the ER. He keeps the keys to our SUV, and when Jack is discharged, he picks us up.

Second, I don't have Kiley and Conrad to help. So I have two bags packed at all times like I've heard pregnant mothers do. One has a change of clothes for Jack and enough clothes for me for three days. The other is my tea, a boiling pot (I bought an extra so I can keep one packed), a mug, bottled water and snacks. I carry extra medicine and other necessary items in my purse at all times.

Third, I need a plan for Juno and Hei Mei if Jack ends up in the hospital. Meghan has agreed to pick Juno up from our house and will put down a huge bowl of cat food and fresh water so Hei Mei can take care of herself.

Finally, we hired a lawn man. Jack mowed our lawn in March getting ready for one of Jeanne's visits, but the oncology nurse cautioned him against this. There are too many possible ways to become infected for Jack to mow. Jack still works outside as much as possible but doesn't mow the lawn anymore.

April 23

Jack isn't waking up this morning. At 8:00 AM I try to wake him to give him his meds. He's delirious. I call William and we get him loaded up in the SUV, and William drives us to the UMMC ER. Just like at Shands, the transport staff comes to take Jack for tests. But quite unlike Shands, Jack tells the transport staff that he will walk back to the ER. "I work here. I know my way. Don't worry about me. I'm heading back to the ER now."

The transport staff returns to the ER bay where I am waiting for Jack. "Where's Mr. Shelton?" he asks.

"With you." I answer.

"He said he was coming back on his own. He didn't?"

Panic seizes me. Immediately I run to the nurses' station and tell them Jack is missing. Then I run outside to make sure he isn't in the street. I run up and down the sidewalks, fear gripping me stronger and stronger with each step. *The idiot – it's his job to care for the patient, not just let him go! Jack was admitted because he's not in his right mind. What's wrong with these people???*

Jack is nowhere to be seen. I run back into the ER to see if he has shown up there. He hasn't.

I know Jack wanted fresh air. This is his stomping ground and he knows the streets because the hospital is adjacent to the building where he works. I go back outside and jog up and down the street looking for Jack.

After what feels like an hour but is only fifteen minutes, Jack comes strutting around the corner of the building, heading towards me and the entrance to the ER.

"Where have you been Jack?" I almost shout but I realize it would be best to try to stay calm.

"I went by my building. I'm okay. No need to worry."

"Well I am NOT okay. You shouldn't be walking around like this."

Jack smiles at me like I'm the crazy one. All I can think is, *He's safe. Don't make a big deal of this. But in the future tell the transport staff that Jack might try this kind of trick and make sure they keep him close.*

Jack has more brain mets. He's in the hospital long enough to get a second round of stereotactic radiosurgery. Even though we've been through this before, this experience is worse. The morning of the procedure three of Jack's colleagues come to the hospital to visit. Jing, of course, is here. When she sees Jack's halo screwed onto his head she can't stop crying.

The surgery helps and Jack's mind starts functioning again. And gratefully, Jack's seizure medicine was changed after his last seizure and Keppra, the new anti-seizure medicine, keeps him from seizing after the procedure.

Jack's room isn't as well equipped as the rooms at Shands, but there is a shower. On the third day Jack is well enough to want to shower. At Shands the towels were available in quantity at any time. At UMMC they are rationed. The shower floor is slightly slanted and since we can't line the floor with towels the way Madison had taught us to do at Shands, Jack slips and pulls his hamstring muscle.

Limping back to his bed, discouragement has taken over. "That's it. I'm never taking a shower in this place again. I don't care if I am here for a month. I'll never step in that shabby stall again."

Is it a purse or an overnight bag?

This may seem like a trivial topic but not if you've lived it. I'm not a high-fashion person and I've never enjoyed carrying a purse. For much of my life I haven't even owned a purse. I stuff my essentials in my pockets, in my glove compartment, or my book bag. A purse is simply too much for me to keep track of and it adds to my already too-heavy workbags. The one item that *will* force me to carry a purse is my cell phone. If whatever I'm wearing and/or already carrying can't provide a secure place for my cell, I'll carry a purse.

The realization has grown slowly that I need to have a purse with me at all times. It started the day Jack was in his wheelchair and we went to outpatient radiation therapy where I left him sitting in the rain to run back to the car for my purse. The Shands Davis Cancer Center had issued Jack a plastic card, like a credit card, that he needed to scan to check in for each of his appointments. But the scanner was at my elbow height, above Jack's comfortable area of reach, so I carried the card. And since he was sitting in a wheel chair, I was carrying his wallet.

Jack's wallet and his patient IMPAC card were just the beginning. As Jack's cancer progresses my purse becomes more and more stuffed. Some days I can't even zip it closed. In addition to what women usually carry in a purse (comb, wallet, pens, checkbooks, lip balm), mine is loaded with essentials:

1. A large post-it pad to make sure I have enough paper at all times to take notes, either about Jack's health or if we are at a medical facility and are given information when I don't have my notebook with me. It's imperative that I write everything down because I can't rely on my memory, which has never been good for details.

2. I was carrying my own toothbrush and toothpaste but

now that we are here in Maryland, I've started carrying two toothbrushes and my dental floss. We spent 27 hours in the ER before being assigned a room, without even the basic needs of water and/or food. I know Jack may be unable to eat or drink because of his medical situation, but there isn't even a water fountain where I can get a drink. Once admitted and assigned a room, I had to ask for personal grooming supplies. So now I carry our own.

3.   My own UMBC ID. If I have my ID I don't have to check in at the registration desk. This is an employee benefit I never expected when I was hired at UMBC.

4.   Washcloths. Jack's physical stability has disintegrated and he spills drinks and drops food more often. I keep washcloths so that he can wipe himself off and still feel proud of his physical appearance.

5.   My vitamins and my prescription drugs, Synthroid and Treximet. In the past I could work with a migraine until I could get home to take my meds but I no longer can do that. First, I might not get home and second, I have to have all systems firing because Jack needs me more than I need myself. The Synthroid is just an assurance in case we have an emergency run to the hospital and I can't get home to grab my overnight bag.

6.   Jack's prescription drugs – two mg crushed Ativan and liquid morphine. Since Jack's seizures I live in constant fear of reoccurrences. The Ativan will help calm the seizure should Jack have another one. The morphine needs no explanation.

7.   Cash. Jack and I have lived on cash for our whole marriage. We use our credit cards only for special occasions. Our usual way to manage our budget is to get a specific amount of money weekly and buy gas, groceries, and entertainment with that set amount of money. We stop spending when it's gone. All of a sudden, I have no way

to get to the bank, which I had previously done every two weeks, to make the withdrawal. Knowing we will need to figure out a way to resupply our cash, I've started being even more frugal, spending only the cash I have to spend. I've turned to the credit cards for most purchases because I am so afraid to find myself without money for a cup of coffee or a bagel should Jack need something from the hospital cafeteria. This wasn't a problem until we came back to Maryland – in Florida Conrad would get money or anything we needed.

8. Travel Wet Ones (antibacterial wipes) and Clorox Wipes. Jack's immune system is compromised so I wipe down all surfaces he comes in contact with. Jack also has to eat when he isn't home, something he loathes. But at least he can wipe his hands before and after meals/snacks.

9. Snacks. Granola Bars to go. I've tried to get Jack to eat the crackers they pass out in the Oncology waiting rooms but he refuses. He will eat a granola bar when it's been too many hours since his last meal. So I carry two or three packs with me at all times.

10. *Clipper Magazine* and a few other coupon books. We go out to eat more than ever and the bills are racking up. I can't say I have the presence of mind to use the coupons, but when I'm home and calm, I know it's a good idea to be able to just grab them once we're settled in an eatery. I suppose if there was one item that I unnecessarily tote along, it's these coupon books.

11. Cards sent to us that I want to respond to, and the cards, postage and pen to write the responses. I can't find time at home to write thank you notes and I don't have the emotional energy to speak to people on the phone, so I carry the cards I want to respond to – only the top priority ones, just two or three at a time. That way if Jack has an unexpected test or we are held up for some unforeseen reason, I have something to occupy my mind.

12. Silverware. I have carried a small pouch with one fork, one spoon and a pair of chopsticks since my second trip to China in 2009. I've added another fork and spoon. At Shands Jack's dinners were served on ceramic plates and in hard plastic bowls, but UMMC serves Jack's food on Styrofoam trays and with plastic forks. Jack and I were shocked – doesn't this hospital know that using Styrofoam is linked to cancer??? How could they deliver a cancer patient's meal with every serving plate made of this crap? At least Jack has a real fork.

13. Lotion, a small eye solution bottle, and a lens case for Jack's contacts. We need the lotion because the radiation has dried Jack's skin out so much it flakes and peels. At various times I lather him up so he feels and looks a little better. The contact lens case and solution is needed just in case we have to rush to the ER and Jack is wearing his contacts.

14. My Kindle – which my sister bought so I don't have to lug around heavy novels, and so that I can read one book after another without having to go either to the library or the bookstore. I also carry a little two by three inch book titled *Encouragement* that Jing sent in one of the care packages. When I feel my deepest moments of despair I pull it out and read one more page.

15. Tea. Almost every day at about 4 PM I boil a cup of water and start my tea drinking for the evening. I only drink Chinese green tea and I only use one packet of leaves per day. Sometimes I pour water over those leaves until there is absolutely no flavor left and I'm drinking straight hot water but that doesn't matter. I need the ritual to help me stay calm. I keep four packets of these loose tea leaves in my purse just in case we end up in the ER. I need at least four because we've never been released from the ER. Once there, Jack is always admitted.

16. Parking passes for the hospital garage. Parking at the hos-

pital in Maryland costs $7 a day unless you're a patient in the Radiation clinic or getting chemotherapy in the oncology clinic. Even though I stay with Jack and we park in his work garage, not at UMMC, I'm obsessed about making sure I have the free parking passes with me. It's impossible to find a place to park in Baltimore. This security is the only way I can ensure smooth access to Jack's doctors and his medical care. So on the days when we park at Jack's work lot, I still take the parking vouchers from the Rad Onc receptionist just in case the day comes when I'm forced to drive to and from the hospital. I know this might happen if Jack ends up as a long-term in-patient. So far I've managed to be with him every night, but my stamina is weakening. I know before long the day might come when I might have to leave him. If that happens, I'll need the extra vouchers.

17. Doctor's business cards and phone numbers. My bag has two external pockets and just keeps accepting more and more and more. In one pocket I slip my cell phone so it won't be lost in the heaps of other things I carry. In the other I keep all the business cards from all the doctors who are part of Jack's team. In Florida I had the numbers for all the Shands clinics and in Maryland I have changed them all to the UMMC contacts. I'm not sure why I've bothered though because at UMMC I'm more likely to be instructed to leave a message but then be informed by an impersonal recorded voice that the mailbox is full. At UMMC I have to email doctors – God forbid I need something when I don't have my computer, access to the internet, and two free hands to type an email. I've asked Dr. Bergoff about this and he claims he has no control over hiring office staff that can manage the volume of phone calls, but from my perspective, this is a *huge* problem.

18. Last but not least, my Daybook. I'm a writer. Some of my entries are just a few words. Some are many pages. I can

go days without opening it up at all. But my Daybook is a part of me I just refuse to leave behind.

It's not a purse. It's not a backpack. It's not an overnight bag. It's my survival bag. And I don't leave home without it.

May 11

Just eleven days after the first discharge, Jack's brain has swelled enough to cause more serious disorientation and lethargy than I've seen before. This morning he is close to a comatose state.

The first time William took us to the hospital, Jack was able to walk. "Okay, left foot forward" I said as I nudged his leg. "Now right foot." But this morning he can't even stand.

William isn't home when I call, so I shift into my backup plan. "Morna. Where are you? I need help. Can you come right away?"

In less than five minutes Morna is running into my house. "I'm up here," I yell down to her, "I have to get Jack to UMMC and he's not able to stand. We have to carry him."

Morna and I somehow manage to get Jack to the top of the landing. Jack has no coordination and can't walk. He almost falls stepping onto the landing – just one step down. We are facing thirteen more steps before we get to the front door, then thirteen more to the street.

Feeling like it is way too dangerous for Jack to try to walk, worried we will lose our grip on him and he will tumble down the stairs, and unable to see any other options, Morna and I are determined to carry Jack down the stairs. We get Jack to sit down on the landing. Morna gets behind him to carry his shoulders and I get in front of him to carry his legs. My cell phone rings just as we were about to start our descent.

"Nancy. It's William. I'm just around the corner. I got your message. I'll be there in two minutes."

Covered in sweat William literally runs to the rescue. Bounding up the stairs two at a time, he slips around me and in front of Morna to hold Jack up by his shoulders. Morna, eleven years younger than I am and much stronger, takes over my job, carrying Jack's lower body down the stairs. I hurry to the SUV, which is in the driveway in the back of our home, and pull it around to the street out front.

William lifts Jack into the passenger's seat and runs around to the driver's side. He breaks every single speed limit between our house and the hospital but does so with no apparent anxiety. He stays calm and cool. "He's going to be okay Nancy. Don't worry. We'll get him there." William is a Vietnam War vet and he knows how to function well under stress.

William is right. We get Jack to the ER before he slips into a coma.

That night, Len comes by to visit. Len and Jack have shared time together over the years in many different spaces, and he knows Jack isn't really here with us even though he is carrying on a conversation.

"Who is sitting next to you Jack?" Len asks.

Jack looks directly at me, then back at Len, and says, "I don't know. That's just some woman. I don't know who she is."

"Jack, don't say that. You know I'm your wife. You know it's me."

"No, I don't know you. Sorry."

Len must see me start to lose control. "Don't Nancy. Don't pressure him. Just go take a walk. I'll stay with him."

While walking through the hospital I keep telling myself the meds will bring Jack back, and they do. But I am shaken. There's no way to explain how it feels to have my husband who I love so much not recognize me.

I realize that someday soon the meds won't be able to bring Jack back. I find solace in the fact that Jack's brain mets will probably kill him before the lung tumor. What a horrible injustice it would be for a man who so loves the water to leave this earth drowning.

As bad as it is, it'll be much better if he can just lose his mind.

In my research I study the effects of creating a positive community in elementary classrooms. It's the teacher's job to make sure that all children know they are welcome in school. That their presence in the classroom makes a positive difference to their peers and to the teacher. That each day the lives of the community members are better because of the contributions individuals make to the environment.

On 8 East at Shands the nurses and staff must have studied the same theory because they made us feel like we were part of a community. They used our names, they talked to us about matters beyond medicine and sickness, and they showed us how much they cared about our lives and our well-being. The nurses welcomed us and made subsequent admissions feel less defeating in their reception of us.

In each of Jack's discharges from Shands the nurses and floor staff made a conscious effort to send us on our way with authentic concern that this time Jack might make it as an outpatient for more than 24 hours. "Mr. Shelton, we love being with you but we'd rather see you at Publix the next time we see you," they'd say. And we could feel they meant it.

At UMMC checking in through the ER is as impersonal as taking a number at the supermarket meat counter and waiting your turn to order your rump roast. And checking out is totally unceremonial. We pack up our belongings, wait for transport, and exit as the strangers we were when we entered.

5-13

Like it has so many times during our marriage, our Anniversary is also Mother's Day. Since moving to Maryland, Jack has planted our vegetable garden on May 13 and this year is no exception.

When Jack first started gardening we were leasing a home surrounded by three acres. When we moved in, the garden, which was at least twenty by forty feet of fenced land with an underground sprinkler system, had been neglected to the point where it took Jack and me two weeks of bushwhacking just to make it possible for Jack to till. For two years we grew more vegetables than I thought was possible without owning a farm. I learned to freeze dry some foods and can others.

Eventually we lived in homes we owned rather than leased, and Jack's gardens became smaller and smaller. But it seems like it doesn't matter, Jack plans and prepares so well that we always have more produce than we can consume without some sort of preserving. Even here in Maryland where his garden is only forty-five square feet Jack's tomatoes, peppers and green beans thrive. It takes Jack all day with many water breaks and rests, but before we share our anniversary dinner he has tucked four tomato plants, four pepper plants and a row of been seeds into the ground. His labor of love is the best anniversary gift I've ever received and he gives it to me year after year.

Longevity

Only once do I tell Jack there's a possible scenario that doesn't include him beating the odds. I ask him to consider making a trip to NY so we can visit Bill and Carol.

"We can spend a week in the Adirondacks, the week between your chemo and the routine testing. That's Memorial Weekend – a good weekend. We can welcome the start of summer like I used to when I was a kid."

"I'd rather not travel during the holiday weekend," Jack says. I'm not surprised at his response because we've never traveled on major holidays unless we had to because of Conrad's sports. But I'm surprised at my own reaction. "Do you mean to tell me that this might be our last summer together and you're not going to take the time to go to Speculator with me?"

Jack turns and looks at me. With great sadness in his voice he says, "So you're not in this for the '5 Year Plan' anymore?"

I'm crushed. He is so convinced he can beat this cancer. There's no doubt his positive attitude makes his days happier and more active. I never should have let my doubt be visible.

Though I never again will mention Jack's longevity, I know inside that each time we do something together that it very well may be the last time.

May 26

This morning I take Jack's temperature as usual, check his blood pressure, and give him his meds. But he doesn't get out of bed.

An hour passes. "Nancy, I feel like something is wrong. Will you please get the thermometer and take my temp again."

"It's 102.5. We have to call Bergoff."

"Yes, and call William too please. I know I need to go in. Let's not wait."

Getting a room at UMMC can take forever. Jack's diagnosis is relatively easy in comparison to his previous ER trips. Today he's put in an ER bay where the staff can close the door and keep others (and hopefully their germs) at a distance.

Only a few minutes pass before Dr. Bergoff walks into Jack's ER bay. Shock registers on Jack's face. It's unmistakable. I'm sure Dr. Bergoff notices it.

"Hi Jack. I'd rather see you in the lab but you don't look so bad. How are you feeling?"

After reading through Jack's chart and talking with Jack, Dr. Bergoff changes his focus to me. "Can I see you outside the room for a minute?"

Once in the hall, his demeanor alarms me. "You know Jack has a DNR, right?"

"Of course, we've spoken about this already."

"I've come over to let you know there's a possibility you will have to act to put the DNR in place if Jack's condition deteriorates."

"What do you mean?" I question.

"Last week I had a patient who also had a DNR. But the emergency room doctors are trained to save lives. They sometimes offer life-saving measures instinctively. If Jack's condition worsens, you may have to stop the medical staff from administering any assistance to him."

No words form in my brain or on my lips.

"Do you understand what I'm telling you, Mrs. Shelton? You may have to physically stand between the doctors and your husband. Can you do that? It's what Jack wants. Can you do it?"

"Yes," I mumble.

"Okay. I know this is difficult and that's why I came to the hospital to see you in person. I am sorry but I know I needed to see you. Call me or have the nurses call me if you need me. Please."

Dr. Bergoff steps into Jack's bay before he leaves. The two men talk about something I can't hear, and even if I could hear what they are talking about I'm sure I wouldn't be able to process it, and then Jack and I are alone. I am cautiously quiet. I don't want Jack to ask me what Dr. Bergoff said to me in the hall. And he doesn't. Maybe he could hear us. Maybe he just doesn't want to know.

We play dress-up for the next three days. Jack has pneumonia. Instead of having people put on protective clothes when they come into Jack's room, we put on protective clothes to leave. It's like déjà vu, but instead of being the oddballs in New Year's Eve regalia we look more like we're dressed for Halloween. We go to the coffee shop. We make laps around the open public spaces inside the hospital. We walk outside after hours and enjoy the relatively quiet sidewalks. We walk anywhere we can as long as we don't expose Jack to more germs.

The infectious disease specialist is friendly. He tells me not to worry about infecting Jack with my germs. "It's counter-productive to worry. He needs you and you come with daily interaction and germ exchange. Just enjoy each other and keep doing what you're doing for each other."

That's the best advice I've heard for a while. I'm going to just enjoy being with Jack and swapping germs until I have no more left in me that he hasn't already acquired.

CHAPTER 19

Finding Humor Wherever I Can

I can't take my eyes off Jack. I don't stare at him when he's look-ing at me, but every chance I get I watch him. I know a day will come soon when he will no longer be with me and I'm trying to burn his physical attributes into my mind so that I will never forget what he looks like, what he feels like, and how his touch feels on my skin. For days I have watched him become thinner and thinner. Even though most of the time I fight not to notice how quickly his body is deteriorating, tonight for some reason, it strikes me as funny to see his skinny little ass.

I was a skinny kid. I was a skinny adolescent, and a skinny young mother. But for some dumb reason, when Conrad was in kindergarten I went on a liquid diet with a mother of one of Con-rad's classmates. In hindsight I was probably just trying to make a friend, so I joined her in her quest to knock off a few pounds. But I didn't have any extra pounds hanging around and the whole diet experience backfired big-time. Years later I realized that by not eating breakfast and lunch for a month I had messed up my metabolism. Since that time, I've had to work to keep my weight in control.

No matter how heavy I got, Jack never ever made me feel fat. When I hit my high mark I was wearing extra-large t-shirts and elastic waist shorts. Conrad was about to start making visits to different universities on baseball scholarship recruiting trips, and I would be the parent who would accompany him on these trips. Fat is the number one prejudice in the United States. I knew the coaches would look at me, a fat mother, jiggling along beside her son who was being evaluated for his athletic prowess. I was out of control, and I really had to do something.

I decided to join a diet center. I was really afraid though because although I was eating too much, I was only eating good foods. I had no interest in eating packaged processed food or taking pills to trick my body. Jack, being the understanding, non-judgmental man he is, agreed to go with me and evaluate the program from a scientist's perspective and as the person who best knew what I could manage. He encouraged me to join, he helped me stick to the diet that required I eat three healthy meals a day, and in 5 months I lost 50 pounds. And because I was young enough, I didn't end up with saggy skin. I've forever been grateful for his support. I vainly want to keep a slender body as long as I can.

Tonight I wish I could laugh out loud with Jack instead of hide behind the bed pillow and keep my humor to myself. Jack, who never had a single fat cell below his waist, has a saggy butt. How worried I was as a young woman that I would have a saggy ass if I waited too long to lose weight. Little did I know that I could stay thin all my life like Jack has done and still end up sagging.

CHAPTER 20

Rapid Decline

Monday, June 4

Conrad has been here for several days helping transport Jack to his radiation treatments and helping me keep the house as happy a place as possible. But Kiley has asked him to go home. She has a doctor's appointment later this week and she wants Conrad to be there with her for it.

Father's Day is coming up soon, and Jack and Conrad have talked about spending time together again then. I know the likelihood of Jack regaining enough strength for all of us to go fishing together is unlikely, but I don't say it to anyone. However, I must have a difficult conversation with Conrad before he leaves tomorrow morning.

This afternoon when Jack is asleep, I ask Conrad to come sit with me on the front steps. I want to be out of the house because I don't want to take a chance that Jack will hear me.

"Conrad, I have to tell you how I'm feeling."

"Okay, Mom, that's why I'm here. What do you want to say?"

"I can't take your father to the hospital anymore. Each time he goes it's worse and worse. I don't need an MRI to tell me he has more brain mets."

"I know it too, Mom. Dad isn't himself. He can't find his words. He's confused. He's frustrated. He tries to hide it but he can't anymore."

"Conrad, I feel like I have two decisions to make. First, if the brain mets start making him unconscious like they did before, I can let him slip into a coma. Or, if his pain increases like it did when we were in Florida and it hit his chest, I can just give him the morphine I have here. I have both liquid and long-acting." I watch Conrad carefully to make sure he's okay as I say these very difficult words – "I just can't make him go back to the hospital anymore."

Conrad looks in my eyes, and I know he's telling me the truth. "Mom, I'm okay with whatever decision you make. That's not my dad in there. I know this is bad. I know you have to make up your own mind on what to do. But you need to know I'm okay with whatever decisions you make."

When Conrad was a toddler he and Jack would lie on the floor every night and "read" *Jack in the Beanstalk.* Each night Jack's rendition of the story changed, but the one thing that remained constant with every reading was Jack's modification of the repeated phrase, "Fee Fi Fo Fum, I'm going to eat me a little one." As soon as he would tell enough of the story and was ready to chase Conrad, Jack would lower his voice, start to roll over, and slowly growl up the words as Conrad squealed, jumped to his feet, and dashed through our apartment giggling, only to be followed by Jack, crawling on his hands and knees chasing his little boy. After a lot of laughing Jack would scoop Conrad up in his hands and roll back down on the floor hugging and tickling his son. The book was finished but not Jack's expressions of love.

I always tease Jack that I'm the one who taught Conrad how to ride a bike, play tennis and throw a baseball, but we three know that Conrad's athleticism is a combination of his genetics blended with my love of sports and the qualities of Jack's personality that come so easily in his son. Take me out to the ball game and I'm happy.

Most babies have rattles and squeaky toys on their blankets. Conrad had a few of those, but mostly he was surrounded by rubber balls, baseballs and tennis balls, and as he grew we added basketballs, soccer balls and footballs to his collection. Conrad loved to be outside as much as I did, and in his preschool days that's where we spent most of our time.

Jack's laid-back way of being complemented the natural skill and love that Conrad had for any sport. Jack and Conrad are patient, kind people who just love to take their time and enjoy each minute of the day.

From Conrad's earliest experiences with organized sports Jack was his most ardent supporter, and also his most unassuming. He has never been the kind of father you so often see in the world of youth sports, living through his son's athletic accomplishments. He's only coached Conrad two seasons, and that was in soccer, which Jack has never even played. Jack prefers not to be around too many kids at once and the only reason he got involved in coaching at all was because he was needed. He's quiet on the sidelines, talks to Conrad about his game performance in private and never brags about his son's accomplishments. And he's always on the sidelines.

When Conrad started playing college ball Jack was most proud, as any father would be. But Jack also stressed the importance of academics. He attended most of the parent/teacher conferences throughout Conrad's years in elementary school, and especially in middle school. Conrad has heard more than once about the time in Jack's life when he had to make a decision to drop out of the walk-on try-outs in college because he knew he couldn't be both a scientist and a baseball player, and that he was most likely to make his mark in life as a scientist.

More than anything sports kept our family focused and together. We shared a common love and Conrad's skill kept us all moving towards a clear destination – the next game. The next win. The next level.

As much as sports played a role in shaping our family, there has always been much more. Weekends at Flagler Beach, skim boarding, boogie boarding and surfing, fishing trips with Pat, Sue, Adam and Kelly, weekends in Tampa with my parents, going wild together on the go-cart track, Jack and Conrad trooping through the archery range with their matching compound bows while I hung out at the truck reading, Fourth of July celebrations, grilling for holidays and normal days, and always taking the time to be together no matter what sort of crazy occurrence was trying to consume our attention.

Through it all, Jack has led by example, showing Conrad what it means to be a fun-loving yet responsible gentleman of the world. Conrad was 25 years old and a student at UF when Jack and I moved to Maryland. The move not only brought Jack and me closer, but it also strengthened the ties between Jack and Conrad. At that time, Conrad composed a note to us that Jack and I have kept tucked away to reread every now and then:

Success? What exactly is success, and how does one know when he or she has been successful? Is it possible that we as Americans have let "Societal Norm" answer this mind-wrenching question? Are we as humans such passive creatures that we allow someone else to tell us what to do to make us happy?

For many years I felt that to be a successful man I had to have more of everything – Money, clothes, watches, etc. Never once did I realize that as an only son born in Pine Rush Apartments, eating plain meals while my father cut down a Christmas Tree out back in the woods because we couldn't afford to buy one, that I was already successful. I was already successful because you wouldn't have it any other way, and you still won't. You have provided for me in ways I can't even express, all things done out of love for me.

God knows that I haven't been the easiest son to raise but this I finally understand – success is happiness. If you are happy, you will in turn be successful.

Mom and Dad, let this be known to you both, I am in every

way extremely grateful for everything you have done. If suc-cess could be measured you would score off the charts.

I Love You.

Thursday, June 7

It's noon before Jack stirs. He's mad at himself because he's "slept half the day away." He still wants to go to the Bass Pro Shop as we had planned – he wants to get the tackle, rods and reels we need for Kiley and Conrad's visit on Father's Day.

Jack showers and dresses while I make breakfast. He moves slowly and it's almost 3:00 PM when we get to the mall. Jack knows exactly what he wants to buy. He walks from one rack of lures to another, sometimes with help from the salesman and sometimes not.

Against my advice Jack has insisted on getting the rod and reel rebuilt that I had when Jack and I met. It's the tackle my former boyfriend picked out for me and taught me how to use when I first moved to Pass-A-Grille. Even the salesman told Jack it was a waste of money, but he insisted. We brought it in the last time we were here, and today when we arrive, we find they were able to replace the eyes on the rod but the reel was returned with a note – "Too old to get parts." So Jack spends time finding a replacement reel similar to the one he can't get rebuilt for me.

He selects two more rods and reels so that we have everything we need to go out as a family – multiple lures, line for the new reels and a tackle box with several insets to sort the lures.

Jack's hiccups persist throughout the day. He has very few peri-ods of rest from them. The only thing that stops them for a while is self-induced vomiting, which he can't do while we're out shopping.

Jack's a slow shopper at the best of times, but today he's almost at a standstill. I worry. I know he needs to eat. Usually he refuses to eat unless he's at home, in a restaurant, or sometimes in our car.

I'm not a shopper. I prefer to go into a store, get what I need, and get out. Jack lingers. He thinks. He makes smart choices. When we shop at the Bass Pro Shop I usually bring a book and sit on the camouflage recliners they have set up and read while I wait for Jack to do his shopping. Today is the same, though I can't focus and read. Jack looks too weak and I am compelled to keep watching out for him. Finally he pushes the cart over to me and shows me everything he wants to buy.

I coax him to sit in the recliner and eat a few granola bars while I go check out. He's willing to do that. I'm stunned. This is the first time Jack has ever eaten in a store since I have known him.

The purchase is over $300.

On our way out of the store, we stop at the Service Desk and buy fishing licenses. One for each of us. Good for one year.

We have dinner in the family room while we watch a few episodes from a television series Jack has found and rented from Netflix – *The Good Wife*. After dinner I serve Jack his gelato. He's become addicted to this high-calorie delight and it's become a routine for us. Dinner with a movie, gelato, then let the dog out and go to bed.

What's not routine is Jack vomiting after enjoying his gelato, but he just asked me to pause the show and I thought it was because he had to pee. Instead he's kneeling over the toilet and brown gelato vomit is in the bowl.

Jack washes his face and comes back to the couch. As we're watching TV, he turns to me and I know to stop the show because he wants to talk. This is another one of our routines – we control the TV instead of the TV controlling us. When one of us wants to say something about the show (or sometimes something unrelated that we just want to talk about) we hit the "Pause" button on the remote and talk.

"I wonder how Kate is going to be with all of this," Jack says.

Confused, with my mind still in the show and thinking I didn't hear him right, I ask, "What did you say?"

"I said, I wonder how Kate is going to be with all this. You know, my cancer."

"Kate. Why do you ask about Kate?" I'd asked Jack to repeat himself but I heard him right the first time.

"She's not as strong as she likes everyone to think. I'm a little worried about her. Didn't she have a pretty hard time of it when her grandmother died? This will be another shock for her."

I can't remember another time when Jack has talked about Kate, and I wonder where his thoughts have come from. Kate is Bill and Carol's youngest child and we haven't seen her in quite a long time. She's at McGill University in Canada and wasn't home when Jack and I last visited Bill and Carol in Speculator. "I'm not too worried about Kate," I respond to Jack, "I'm more concerned about Bryan and Bethany. They just lost their Uncle Kenny not too long ago and they were really close."

I restart the show.

Not too many minutes pass before Jack again starts a conversation. "I'd like to get together with Mike and Cathy. I'd like to talk to Mike." Mike and Cathy are Kiley's parents, and Mike is a preacher at a church in the Panama City area.

I assure Jack that I'll contact them and see if they can fit in a visit. Jack says that he can even talk on the phone, and gently, looking at me as he talks, says, "At the expense of sounding morbid, I'd like Mike to say a few words for me."

I'm shocked and I don't know what to say, but know I need to say something. So I tell Jack I'll get in touch with Cathy and see if we can get together. Before I restart *The Good Wife*, I'm happy to tell Jack, "If it helps at all, I've already spoken to Mike and he's agreed to speak for you."

"Good. Thank you."

Panic rises in my chest. My brain races looking for words that

I know I must speak. I restart the show but I can't watch TV at this moment.

I hit the "Pause" button again, and look at Jack. "It's my turn honey." I smile, hoping a smile can somehow make a sad moment less sad.

Jack looks over at me, his eyes as expressive as they have always been. Hiccups jarring his body at regular intervals.

"At the expense of me sounding morbid, is it okay with you if you're cremated?" I'm speaking as normally as possible in spite of the restriction I feel in my throat and the pain I feel in my heart.

"Yes." is his simple response. It gives me strength to continue.

"And I thought I would have a service for you at Crystal River."

"That would be nice." Jack says this as he turns his head towards the television. I take that as my cue, and hit the "Play" button on the control. The noise from the television fills the room. I don't hit pause again until the show is over.

If an angel appears in my family room and wants to play a trading game with me offering Jack's life for a retelling of the show I am watching, I wouldn't be able to conjure up one single event in the plot. The conversation I just had with Jack reveals to him that I know he is dying. He knows I have been making plans and talking to people about his inevitable death and that I have not had these conversations with him. Not until tonight. My body feels cold. My mind feels heavy. I know I have to somehow thaw out and find strength to support Jack as he continues his fight but I don't know how I will do it. I hide under my afghan. Somehow I keep my usual routine and at a slow moment in the show, I reach out and rest my hand on Jack and say, "Have I told you lately that I love you?" My voice is strong and Jack smiles. His smile gives me strength.

"I love you too."

Tonight, like every night after we finish watching TV, when Jack climbs the stairs I watch him. It's a good thing Vince will be here tomorrow to install the handrails. We have rails on one side of the staircases but Jack needs to be able to grip with both hands. He doesn't have the strength to climb tonight.

Every step is a laborious process. He takes a few steps, leans forward, rests, and then continues for a few more steps.

When he gets to the top of the stairs leading from the family room I hold my breath. There's no handrail for the uppermost four stairs and I'm so afraid he will lose his balance. He doesn't. Pulling himself up using the doorway, he turns the corner at the landing.

When he's entirely in the living room, I breathe again. Living in a three-level home is a challenge at times but it's even more so for Jack right now.

Once on the main floor, I load the dishwasher while Jack gets the Netflix DVD ready for the mail.

He lets Juno out the front door and before too long we're ready to go up to our bedroom.

Again I watch Jack. I sit on the couch, trying to seem normal. I don't want to stand behind him because I want him to think I have confidence in his ability to manage himself. Again he's leaning forward his whole way up, using the stairs above him to help him balance and to give himself time to rest.

I wonder how long he's going to be able to make this climb.

CHAPTER 21

Only Recline

Friday, June 8

I feel bumping and rocking in my sleep. I roll over and the rocking increases. In a state of semi-consciousness, I roll over on my back and reach my left arm out to rest it on Jack. In that second before my new reality takes over, I think, *Jack must be getting ready for work.* I barely complete the thought before my mind registers and I'm jolted into panic. *Jack is not getting ready for work. He's not in the bed. Juno is rocking my bed with her head and moving her body in an anxious way. Where's Jack?*

As I jump out of bed Juno starts hurrying towards the bedroom door. I understand. I must follow her. I do. Juno leads me directly to Jack. He's in the bathroom, sitting on the toilet, holding onto the vanity with his left hand and gripping his Gatorade bottle in his right hand. It's grape Gatorade this morning. Dark purple.

"I can't get up," Jack says as I rush in to the room. "I can't get up. I can't finish shitting. I don't know what I'm doing. I can't get up." Jack's body seems like it's trying to stand. I see him lurch up but his legs don't work and he stays sitting on the toilet. I have no idea what is happening, but whatever it is, it's not good.

"It's okay," I say, reaching out to him and gently rubbing his back. I hope my touch will register as a calm feeling and that Jack's brain will re-engage.

Jack and I have slept naked with each other our entire lives together. Lately he's been sleeping in his shirt, or sometimes even a sweatshirt, because he's so cold. Even turning up the heat in our waterbed has not kept him warm enough.

Last night he wore his old *Shadracks* shirt to bed. It's one of the old white ones. We each have one but Jack steals mine so really, he has two and both are threadbare at the neck. I've seen Jack in this shirt so much it brings me comfort that he is wearing it now. He's still Jack. Still a beach boy. Still mine.

"You're okay, honey. I'll help you." I take the Gatorade bottle out of his hand and set it on the sink. Then I wad a bunch of toilet paper and, as I did for Conrad when he was a child, I wipe Jack to assure him he has not made a mess. There are no feces in the toilet bowl. He has not moved his bowels, though he's confused and thinks he has. I stand in front of Jack, steady him by holding both his hands in mine, and help him rise off the toilet.

This is worse than ever. Jack had to have help walking back in Florida when the bone mets landed him bedridden, but he's been fully mobile for months. And even then, when he started PT and got back on his feet, he was steadier than he is this morning.

Holding onto Jack, my left hand holding his left hand, my right arm around his waist, I guide him into our bedroom and help him lower himself onto the side of our bed. He has control when I guide him. He's able to balance on the edge of our waterbed, not falling backwards onto the mattress. I sit beside him, rubbing his back, letting him know he's okay.

It's 7:30 AM. Jack says, "I'm tired."

"Yes, honey, you should lie back down. But before you do, you should take your meds. It's only a half hour before you need them and this way I won't have to wake you."

"First help me put my jeans on."

I guide Jack's feet into his jeans, help him stand, and with his weight only gently leaning towards me, I zip his fly, button his jeans, and buckle his belt. I help him ease back down onto the side of our bed.

I return to the bathroom for Jack's Gatorade. I hand him the Gatorade and cross the bedroom to the dresser to get his meds.

I'm back with Jack in just seconds. As I try to hand him his meds, he says, "I don't want them."

I re-explain. "It's so close to 8 AM. You should take the meds now so you can sleep."

Again, Jack repeats, "I don't want them."

Jack has never refused his meds. Not one single time since Terrible Tuesday has he been difficult about anything so I know his brain is completely confused. And it's more than just not being able to go to the bathroom or navigate back to the bedroom. I'm not sure what to do so I raise my voice a little and say, "You need to take your meds."

Jack looks up at me and says nothing. I put his Keppra in is mouth. He spits it back out. I catch the pill before it falls. "Stop this. You need to take your medicine." I feel horrible being so stern.

Resting his left arm on his left knee, with the Gatorade in his hand, Jack looks at me and with defiance in his voice, says, "Okay. Just tell me what you want me to do and I'll do it."

Calmly, I say, "I want you to take your medicine. Here, I'll give you one pill at a time, you use your Gatorade and just take the meds." I hand Jack his pills and he takes them. Relieved, I sit down next to him and start rubbing his back again.

Jack turns to me. His voice is quiet. "You are being mean to me." I feel so sad I want to cry, but I can't. I keep rubbing his back. "I'm not being mean, Jack, I'm just making sure you have your meds so you can rest and not have another seizure." We sit together like this for a few minutes while Jack finishes his Gatorade. Then he hands me the empty bottle, I set it aside, and help him get back in bed. I pull the covers up to keep him warm. Almost instantly he's asleep.

Since Jack woke so late yesterday, I know he'll sleep for a while this morning. We have no chairs in our bedroom, and instead of sitting on the bed I decide to move the Papasan chair from my study into the bedroom so I can be near Jack. I don't want to just rely on the baby monitor to hear him. I want to be physically close to him.

I sit in my chair and watch Jack breathe. Last night's conversation replays in my mind. I know without a doubt that Jack is worse than I have ever seen him, worse even than when he didn't know who I was when I was sitting next to him in the ER the second time we had to go to UMMC, the day he couldn't walk downstairs and William and Morna had to carry him. Worse than when he cried out in pain from his hip and his chest pain back when we were in Florida. Now I'm not sure his mind can even register pain.

Before I settle in to read, I pick up the phone. "Hi Kiley. I know I've called you at least three times to tell you I don't think Jack will make it another day, but this time I'm sure. Please talk to Conrad and see if he or both of you want to come up immediately. You need to get the first flight you can if you want to see Jack."

When I push the "Off" button on the phone I stare at the handset for several minutes. How unfair this is to Kiley. She and Jack have a special relationship that I can't even understand so I surely can't explain. I'm sure her pain is great, but it's her I turn to for strength. I feel so grateful Conrad has her to lean on. I hope she can feel how much of a difference she has made in our little family.

Mitch Rapp has stopped all the terrorists he can until his reappearance in a newly released book. Carol and Meghan have been helping me keep a supply of reading on hand. I select one of Meghan's books, Picoult's *House Rules*.

I set the chair in front of the window directly next to Jack, position my cell phone on the edge of the chair within immediate reach, and start reading.

What do people who do not read do to escape the pain and anguish in real time? In life? In death? Jack is dying. I know it but I turn to my book and act like I can just read and all will be fine. All of Picoult's books end with a totally unexpected twist. Maybe if I keep reading long enough Jack's fight with cancer will take an unexpected turn from a quickly approaching end to a slow, rejoicing recovery.

About 9:00 AM I get a text from Vince. He's on his way with all the supplies he needs to install the handrails. I grab the baby monitor and head down to the family room. Vince arrives just as I'm opening the gate for him so he can park his trailer in the driveway. It's a relief to see him and it's not just because I know Jack will have an easier time climbing the stairs once the handrails are installed.

"Vince, Jack is still sleeping. He was not well this morning at all. I don't know how long he'll sleep. Do you mind starting on the family room stairs just to keep the noise an extra floor away?"

"Would it be better if I wait?" Vince asks. "I don't have to do this today. Or I can come back later."

"No, I need the railings up. Yesterday Jack slept until well after noon, and he was weak last night. I'd rather have the noise and the handrails than quiet without. But thanks." What I don't say is equally as important – *I need you here. I don't want to be alone.*

Vince gets started and I head back upstairs to be with Jack. When Carol sent her usual text this morning I told her Jack was disoriented but that I had gotten him settled back in bed to sleep more. As I tried to read, Carol and I continued texting. Concern grows in me as I explain how desperate I feel. I had just sent Conrad home two days ago because Kiley needed him but I really need him to be here with me.

At 10:00 Jack suddenly sits upright in the bed and starts yelling. "OH MY GOD. MAKE IT STOP. IT HURTS. MAKE IT STOP. LET ME DIE. IT HURTS." Clutching his chest he thrusts himself towards the middle of our bed.

I jump out of the chair. "Where does it hurt? Jack, What's the pain? Is it something new?"

Jack rocks back and forth on the bed, his arms bent, his left hand holding his right hand against his chest.

I measure out a dose of liquid morphine. Touching Jack on the shoulder, I gently ease him toward me. "Here's your morphine. I have it all ready." Jack allows me to slip the meds in his mouth. He stops yelling but continues to rock back and forth.

"Here, honey. Take this too. It's another 60 mg of slow release."

As Jack calms, I situate him back in bed. Gently stroking his forehead, I use as soothing a voice as I can. "It won't take long. You'll be okay. I'm going to give you another bit of the liquid morphine, just to help until the long-acting kicks in."

I stroke Jack's face until his breathing changes and I know he's resting. Then I sit in the chair and cry. Silently.

Realizing I don't want to be alone, I type a text to Carol, "Is there any way you can come down? Just until I can get Conrad back up here. I understand if you can't." I stare at the text. It's June 8. Carol's family is always together and busy in the summer. I can't ask her to come down. I don't send the text.

Exactly six minutes later, the phone rings. I push the "Talk" button before the first ring finishes. I don't want Jack to wake up until the morphine has a chance to get into his system.

"Hello," I whisper into the phone.

"If I leave by noon, I can get to your house by about eight tonight. Do you want me to come down?"

I can't believe it. It's as if I sent the text. I look at my phone. No, I didn't. Carol just knows I need her. "Please."

"Kate will be with me. Is that okay? She's going to help me drive."

"Of course. Thanks Carol. I can't talk. I don't want Jack to wake up. I don't want to leave his side."

"Okay, but just listen for a minute. Don't let Jack sleep through taking his meds. Make sure and wake him. He needs the pain medication. Okay. I'll see you soon."

"Okay," I whisper, and push the "Talk" button again to hang up the phone. Tears just gush out of my eyes. My nose burns. I can't control my breathing. I'm afraid I'll make noise and wake Jack.

It takes a long time for me to calm down. When I do, I quietly sneak out of the bedroom to go check on Vince. I'm sure he heard Jack yell, and it must be hard for him. Vince's own mother is a cancer patient. His emotions must be tangled up in a knot too. Yet he's willing to be here to help Jack and me. We're so lucky to have such good friends. Again Vince wants to make sure he should keep working. The drill is loud, as is the saw. I ask him to get all the handrails up if he can. He assures me he'll do his best.

I spend the day next to Jack. Several times at irregular intervals Jack's hand raises and trembles. I know he's seizing. I know the tumors and edema are taking over his brain. Every second Jack breathes more and more of his brain is destroyed. I know he will never speak to me again. I doubt he will ever get out of bed again.

I read as much as I can but mostly I just sit in the chair and watch Jack. I'm tired. I rest my book on my chest and close my eyes.

When I wake up it's 4:15 PM and I realize Jack still has not stirred, I know for sure he's dying. But somehow, death is no longer an unwelcomed stranger, it's not some unknown entity, or a fear that has crept into every one of my days since Jack's cancer hit. At this moment I understand it. Death is a part of life that needs to be embraced. It needs to be welcomed. It is necessary. It is the next thing for Jack to do. Without fear. Without regret. Without resistance. We need to welcome death as it arrives.

I'm jolted out of my thoughts when I hear the drill. Vince is still working on the railings. *I must have missed Meghan* I think. She was supposed to come over after she finished teaching.

Vince is working on the railing leading from the main floor up to our bedrooms. "Wow. This looks great. Thanks so much Vince," I say as I emerge from the bedroom.

When I get to the main floor, I see Meghan. She's waited for me. We were supposed to have a salad together but she had a sandwich instead – good thing, because I'm not hungry and I don't want to be in the kitchen.

Meghan and I go down to the family room. I don't want to take a chance that my voice will disturb Jack.

"Can I do anything for you, Nancy?"

"No, Meghan, thanks. There's just nothing we can do."

"Do you want me to go get anything from the store for when your sister gets here?"

"No, we'll just order from Hunan Joy if Kate and Carol haven't eaten when they get here."

Meghan is telling me about her last day at work – the school year has drawn to a close. We hear Jack's breathing change. I turn the monitor up so I'm sure to know if Jack wakes.

Our conversation switches to the cookout we had planned for Memorial Day that we were trying to reschedule. I realize this is one dinner we will never share. "I'm losing him Meghan."

"You can't be sure. He's bounced back so many times. He might again."

"Yes," I say, running my hands through my hair to relieve the tension I feel in my heart.

The monitor is the next noise we hear. Jack's started hiccupping. His breathing is changing again. It sounds like he's wheezing. I hug Meghan and we go upstairs.

Vince is putting the finishing touches on the railings. I thank them both and go to my bedroom to be with Jack.

As I watch Jack, I'm more and more positive he's dying. The

house is quiet. I start to worry about my decision not to call the paramedics and to let Jack die at home. In Florida I could have called Hospice to make sure I'm okay but I'm not in Florida.

I dial Dr. Bergoff's office number. I get his machine. I wait on the line to leave a message but hear a robotic, "This mailbox is full." I stare at the phone in disbelief. How can an oncologist have such shitty office management that I can't even leave a message? I'm not calling a million numbers to try to connect to a doctor. I don't have the time, the energy or the ability to talk that much.

My second call is to Steve, Jack's neurologist and our friend. He answers immediately.

"Steve, I'm sorry to bother you but I need help."

"What can I do? Just name it."

"Jack is dying. I need to know if I'll be in legal trouble if I don't call an ambulance."

"Oh Nancy, I'm so sorry."

"Thanks Steve. I just need to know if I can just stay home with Jack and let him die in peace."

"This is a very personal decision. Jack can't make it. You are the next person to make the decision. There is no legal reason you need to call an ambulance. If you think Jack would want to die at home, that is your choice."

At 7 PM a text beeps in from Carol. "Make sure you give Jack his 8 PM meds. Wake him if you have to."

I let Jack sleep. I can't make myself disturb him. He's peaceful and I'm letting him stay that way.

I'm curled in the Papasan chair when Kate and Carol arrive at 8:30 PM. They break the silence in my home. Though the situation is somber, their conversation is light-hearted. I set my monitor up on the stereo downstairs in the living room so we can talk but I can still hear if Jack needs me.

It's a relief to discuss traffic and to listen to Kate and Carol quip back and forth about who's a better driver. We order Chinese food, which Kate gladly goes to pick up because they drove straight through dinnertime. We're just sitting down to eat when a loud moaning sound is transmitted through the baby monitor.

Jack's cries are loud and strong. I don't need the monitor to hear him. Carol and I fly up the stairs. When I approach the bed, I see fear in Jack's eyes. He can't speak. The noise he is making is similar to the noise he made during his first seizure. His hands are pushing at the sides of his forehead. He has wet his pants so I quickly remove them and get the urinal but he doesn't need it anymore. I position a hospital chuck under him and pull our comforter back over him to keep him warm.

"Nancy, get Jack's meds and give him morphine right now. He's in pain. He needs it."

Jack spits out his pills, just like this morning. I switch to liquid morphine and put it along the side of his mouth as Carol instructs. When he stops moaning, I put the Keppra in his mouth again. Again he spits it out.

Jack's eyes are wide open – unnaturally so – as he looks back and forth from me to Carol. He's still holding his head the same way we all hold our heads when we have a wicked headache. Finally he rests his eyes on Carol. Jack is calming and Carol steps closer to him. She takes his hand and starts talking to him. "Jack, how are you doing? You don't look so great. You need your meds. They will make you feel better and take some of the pain away. Just let Nancy give them to you."

It's clear to me that Jack understands. His eyes travel to me and I hold my hand on the side of his face and say, "Okay, Jack, just swallow your pills. I'll put them there for you."

I only give Jack the Keppra and the morphine – none of his other meds. His breathing returns to normal and he closes his eyes.

"He knew you would come. He's been waiting for you to get

here. Now that he knows you are here he can let go. He didn't want me to be alone. He's going to die tonight. I'm staying here but you can go finish dinner with Kate."

I can hear Carol and Kate cleaning up the dinner. I realize that the baby monitor is on and that Kate heard everything, all of Jack's cries and moans, all of our words. How odd that Jack seemed to know this in advance – last night he was worried about how Kate would manage his death even before we knew that Kate would be here with us.

Kate comes up to say good night before she heads to the family room which serves as our second guest room, complete with an air mattress and private bathroom.

When Carol comes in to talk, I climb on the bed, sitting next to Jack so Carol can sit in the chair. "I told you that you should have woken Jack up to give him his meds," she admonishes me.

"You're probably right, but I just couldn't disturb him. He's been seizing all day and I honestly wasn't sure he would even regain consciousness at all. He keeps fighting back. But I think his fight is gone."

"You might be right. Jack is one of the nicest people I've ever met in my life and I'm sure he wants to take care of you as much as he can. If he had to wait and be in pain until I could get here so you're not alone, he would do it."

Carol takes Jack's hand again and starts talking to him. "When you see Bee tonight tell her I miss her. Tell your father 'Hi' even though I never met him, I'm sure he's a good man."

CHAPTER 22

Death

Saturday, June 9

At 1:00 AM I send Carol to bed. I strip, climb into bed with Jack, feeling his skin from my waist down and slipping my hand under his shirt so I can rub his bare chest. Jack's hand comes up to my arm, and he cradles my arm in his hand as he has done so many times.

I want to talk to Jack before it's too late, to I tell him how much I love him. "You have taught me how to be a good person by being that person – a man who doesn't criticize people, who finds good in even the most difficult situations, who truly cares for and helps his friends. You have financially provided for me for 35 years, nursed me when I was sick, taught me how to love with a fierce passion, and led me into a professional world where I've been successful only because of your constant support."

I know the end is near and I need to let Jack know I have loved him more than anything in this world. I need to say the words even though he can't speak back to me. "Thank you for my life, for our lives, for your care and guidance, for our son."

I tell him I'm so much a better person because of my life with him. "Conrad is a fine, intelligent, sensitive man because you are his father." I tell Jack that when he sees his own father I want Jack to tell him that I'm sorry I never got to meet him. "And when you see Adam, tell him I'm still mad at him for killing himself." When I say this, Jack squeezes my hand.

I stop talking, just sensing Jack's presence beside me. I know this is the last time I will feel this intimacy. I reach down and touch every part of Jack's body. I rub my hand over his arms and legs, feeling his thick curly hair I have loved for so many years. I hold his penis in my hand, soft and warm. I gently move my fingertips across his forehead, cheeks and neck the way he has always loved me to touch him. Then I snuggle as close to him as possible and lie there listening to him breath.

Jack's breathing changes. It sounds heavy. And slow. It's more and more irregular.

I don't know why I think of this one event when Jack is dying but maybe it's because I am so relieved his brain mets are killing him and not his lungs filling with fluid. He's not going to drown. No man who was so great a swimmer, who so loved his life as a Florida Beach Boy should drown in his own body fluids.

I don't even know for sure exactly how lung cancer patients die. All I know is that when our friend, Dr. Zam, died of lung cancer that presented similarly to how Jack's presented, his wife told us that Dr. Zam had essentially drowned. She said she could hear his lungs fill with fluid he could not extract.

Whatever the reason for my fear, it's real. Over these last few weeks I can't get one specific memory out of my mind.

Jack, Pat, Sue, and I were offshore in the Gulf of Mexico in Pat's Mako. It was 1977. We weren't even married yet. We had planned a day of fishing and, as usual, Jack, Sue and Pat were also going to dive.

After we had gotten so far offshore I couldn't even see land, in the usual cocky way Pat and Jack always try to one-up each other, Pat said, "Jack, dive on down there and check the bottom to see if this is a good place to drop our lines."

Jack started walking towards his SCUBA gear.

"You don't need that – according to the Loran it's only fifty-two feet."

I didn't know a lot about fishing, but I knew fifty-two feet was too deep to free dive.

"No problem Captain," he said as he grabbed his flippers, put them on, and slipped off the side of the boat with his mask in hand. Jack was accepting the dare.

Jack was gone for what felt like an eternity. I kept staring at the place by the boat where he went down. I'd quickly glance at Pat to see if he was nervous and then return my gaze to the water.

It was every bit of three minutes before Jack came popping back up out of the Gulf. I was so new to this lifestyle I didn't even realize Jack wouldn't come back up where he went down – he would be several feet away.

Jack swam beside the boat, raised his hands while calling Pat. "Hey Captain Pat. This isn't a good place to fish. Sandy bottom." As he said those words, he opened his hands and let the wet, loose sand run down his palms to his wrists, streaking down the exposed parts of his arms.

At 2:45 AM, Jack's breathing changes again. He's struggling more. I know I must get out of bed, I must get Carol, I must face that this is the end. I reluctantly leave Jack's side, put on a few clothes, and wake my sister.

Seconds later I return to the room and again climb on the bed with Jack. Carol is talking to him. I'm sitting next to him and Jack reaches over and puts his hand on my leg. He starts to move around and at one point suddenly sits up.

When he lies back down, I straddle him, take his face in my hands and move his head so that our eyes meet. Jack reaches up and puts his hand on my chest. I take Jack's hands in mine and hold them. Gently.

Jack struggles for air. He has stopped breathing but I know he's not gone. I keep holding his hands in one of my hands, and I gently close his eyes. It's untrue that you can close a person's eyes after he dies and I know this. I will need Jack to seem as if he is sleeping once he has left me.

Three minutes pass. It is exactly 3:00 AM. Jack takes one final gasping breath.

In the split second between Jack's life and his death I hold his hands in mine and feel all the love of 35 years pass easily and peacefully between us.

Epilogue

I can only try to remember my first year and a half after Jack died. I have some artifacts, some emails, a few pictures, but I quit writing. I can piece some things together but the pieces never measure up to a whole.

As I have written in this memoir, my family and friends were extremely supportive during the 5 months, 13 days Jack was fighting his cancer. That support continued directly after his death.

My first year was what I refer to as my "year of flight" when I traveled between Maryland, New York and Florida at a pace that would make a truck driver look stationary. I traveled to the United Kingdom with Pandora. I spent a week in the mountains of Tennessee with Conrad.

I took Juno everywhere I could, especially to New York where we would stay at Carol and Bill's for weeks at a time and Juno could run, play and swim with Carol's dog. The long trips on the road were hard on Juno because she couldn't manage to get comfortable on the back seat of the Benz. Though it broke my heart to let it go, I needed to be able to travel with my dog, so I traded in my beloved little car and purchased an SUV.

Juno's love and attention was one of the few constants in my life. Many days she was the only living being I would talk to. When I would lie in bed, unable to sleep, her snoring kept me company. Her need to be fed, walked and let out each morning were often the only scheduled tasks I attended to.

I stopped cooking and started drinking. Unless Meghan was coming for dinner I'd just throw lettuce and cucumbers in a bowl, call it a salad and call that dinner. Meghan knew what a mess I was and made herself a regular Thursday night guest whenever I was in Maryland. So I cooked once a week. I refused to let my house seem lived in, putting everything away with some sort of compulsive need I have never had in my life. I slept only in bits and spurts, usually just a few hours at a time.

I quit reading too. My most serene moments were those when I was engaged in manual labor. I learned from my neighbors Monica and Kyle how to fix the cracks in the plaster and with Vince's help, I finally finished the family room remodeling Jack and I had started seven years earlier. Then with an equal measure of passion I attacked the dining room and painted that room with another friend, Donna. My house almost became a place I could manage to inhabit for more than a few consecutive nights. Almost. So I turned my sights on the kitchen. Mikey gutted the old and rebuilt an entirely new kitchen for me. Floor to ceiling.

And I re-taught myself how to cry. It took music, loud music that was not part of Jack's and my relationship. Lyrics that made me so sad I would weep for hours.

Our society deals very poorly with the grief one experiences in losing a life partner to death. After a year many people didn't even offer the usual, "Oh, I'm sorry," when, for whatever reason, I mentioned that I "lost" my husband. Some people even became visibly upset if Jack's name came up in conversation. Others quickly tried to divert the topic away from any mention of him.

A number of friends just stopped contacting me. Occasional communications were sometimes worded so that I knew my pre-ordered response was to say, "Oh, I'm well, thanks," which was almost always a blatant lie.

People kindly offered advice that I would soon "find a new normal" or "move on" or even "get over it." None of these platitudes were what I felt was happening to me. I was, quite simply, trying to figure out how to live when all I really felt was *nothing*. Joan Didion calls this the experience of "meaninglessness itself."

At the same time I felt like I was struggling to find a way to hide my grief from the people who were uncomfortable with my weakness, there were other people who never gave up on me. My relationships with those people have flourished. It is a complicated process to rebuild your life after such a terrible loss, and what is built back is not the same as what was destroyed. And it takes a lot longer than one year.

My relationship with Conrad has been the single most important one of all. Three months after Jack's death, Kiley moved out and on what would have been Jack's 59th birthday, December 20, 2012, they were divorced. The trauma this caused for both Conrad and me strengthened what was already a very strong relationship. Kiley's absence in our lives forced me to stop thinking so much about my own loss and start thinking about how much Conrad had lost. I would sit and wonder how in the hell he was going to survive losing his father and his wife in such a short period of time, telling myself that might be worse than me losing a husband and a daughter-in-law. Logically I knew there was no comparing such things, but it took me quite a long time to think logically again.

Something very special happens when a family of four reduces suddenly to a family of two, if the two left are able to provide emotional support for each other. Throughout the worst of our grief, we each had a depth of understanding that needed no words, no explanation, no overt attention. We both just knew so much of what the other was feeling that that knowledge itself in some way made each of us feel not so much alone.

Eventually I returned to work, teaching my regular courses at UMBC and meeting with doctoral students on a somewhat regular schedule.

The book contract Bess and I had secured in November 2011 had to either be honored or dissolved. Bess had, unfortunately, hit a rough patch in her life too, and she couldn't manage the project on her own. We had to either write or let all our previous work swirl down the drain.

But my brain had been injured by the stress of Jack's illness and death. Grief continued to impair me cognitively. I had to find a way to heal. I didn't know where to start or what to do.

Finally, quite by accident, I realized that if I was near Bess physically, she could talk and I could write. The partnership we've always shared as researchers took on a completely new quality the second year after Jack died. Instead of two minds working together in harmony with each other, challenging each other in ways that made us both qualitatively better thinkers, we put our two minds together to barely make one mind. One plus one equaled less than one.

Day after day I would drive to Bess's house and for hours we'd work. My thinking finally got strong enough to write at home, but only after Bess and I had discussed in depth what I needed to write, or revise, and only if she was available by phone to help pull me out if I got stuck. Our completed manuscript was finally submitted April 9, 2014 and was published in November 2014, in time for our major professional conference, the National Council of Teachers of English (NCTE).

The same month Bess and I submitted our manuscript to Routledge Press I started running. Nothing helped my emotional healing the way running did. One of Jack's colleagues, Nick, sent me an email on April 7, 2014 to let me know he was running the 5K in the Maryland 5K and Half Marathon. The run is sponsored by the Greenebaum Cancer Center at UMMC and the funds raised are designated for cancer research at UMB. Nick was running for Jack. He invited me to either join him, come cheer him on, or neither. He just wanted me to know he was organizing a team, he was running for Jack, and that I was welcome.

That night I contacted my friend in Gainesville, Lisa, who I had run with for a very brief time back when we were both classroom teachers together at Duval Elementary School. Those two years running with Lisa were the only time I have ever enjoyed the sport. Lisa assured me that I could meet this challenge, and that she would fly up to Maryland and run with me. Lisa and I registered for the race. Not the 5K but the half marathon.

I only had one month to train. Another friend, Carla (Mikey's wife) helped me. Her words were honest and encouraging. "Nancy, you don't have enough time to really hurt yourself. I know you. I can't tell you not to do this. But after this race, you have to start over and be smart and train right."

The truth was that I wanted to feel pain even though my pain was nothing like Jack's. I had chosen this race. He had not chosen lung cancer. Every time I was out there training for the run, if I thought I might not make it, I visualized Jack. Bedridden. Unable to move his legs. Unable to walk. Unable to even sit in his wheelchair comfortably. Then I would visualize him back at work, smiling for a picture at the elevator his first day back, him planting our garden on our anniversary less than a month before he died. And I kept running.

On May 12, just one day before what would have been Jack's and my 36th wedding anniversary, wearing bib number 513, I ran my first half marathon. Lisa and Carla spent their Mother's Day weekend helping me find some way to make it through an incredible feat. The three of us crossed the finish line together in just under three hours.

The symbolism was not hidden. If I could endure the physical challenge and pain and run 13.1 miles in my first race ever, I could endure the emotional challenge of living without Jack physically present in my life.

Shortly after I started training for the half marathon, I started writing again. But I couldn't write about my present life. I could only write about Jack. And so this book began to take shape. I found purpose in my days. I had a story to tell, and it was a story I hoped might help others find the strength to face whatever challenges were present in their lives. The strength to love with a passion that does not die. The strength to live with the hope that each sunrise will awaken dreams, purpose, and life from deep within oneself.

I'm finding that strength. On January 18, 2015 Lisa and I ran together again. She's a much more accomplished runner than I am, but I took Carla's advice, trained more intelligently, and ran my second half marathon in Key West. We rented an attic space (billed as an apartment) and spent a long weekend together. Lisa and her husband, Dave, brought three bicycles, and I brought a desire to play. For the first time since Terrible Tuesday, I had several days of nothing but nonstop fun. We rode the bikes all over Key West. We went to Papa Joe's and drank draft beer. We went to Margaretville and drank… of course… Margaritas. We went to breakfast at Pepe's Café, lunch at the Half Shell Raw Bar, and dinner at Michael's Restaurant. We rode our bikes to Zachary Taylor's Historic State Park, toured the park, and then rode to South Beach. After the race, we drank beer and danced in the street. We laughed. We cried. We lived.

For over two years every single day I had to repeat this mantra just to get myself out of bed – "Jack died, you didn't. Get up and live." As this book goes to press I can honestly say I'm on the road headed back to happiness. I've learned how to do the things Jack always did – mow the lawn, take out the garbage (on the right day), plant and maintain a vegetable garden, wash the car, feed the animals, grocery shop, and even "man" the grill. When I'm home, I've become much more routine in my living, knowing that the example Jack set was one I can and should follow. I've been held by another man and felt good from my head to my toes. I've managed to survive financially, present at an international writing conference in Paris, France, get promoted to Full Professor, and write this book. I'm up and living again.

When I awoke the morning of April 7, 2015, I was only too aware that I had been granted more life than Jack, because I was the exact age he was on June 9, 2012, when he died. It was one of the hardest dates I had to face alone. But I had already learned that the best approach for me is to plan something for these special dates so that I'm not moping around the house where sadness can swallow me up in one quick gulp.

In preparation for this date, I searched for and joined a local widow/widowers group. That afternoon I dressed in my best jeans and a stunning sweater and joined a fabulous group of people for happy hour at the bar where Jack and I used to go to watch the Gators play football.

The stuffed bear Jack's colleagues at UMB sent to him in one of his care packages never did capture his smell, but it has a new purpose. It sits on my bed as an eternal reminder of the playfulness that was so much a part of Jack's personality and his relationship with the people in his lab, celebrating his conscious decision to live as happy a life as possible and to help those around him find a little fun in every day.

I surround myself with people who help me feel positive about myself. Oddly enough, one of those people is Jing, Jack's research colleague. She and I have developed a friendship that we didn't have when Jack was alive and healthy. It's a friendship that is lasting, one that for me feels like we are sisters-in-law, with a special love for Jack that will never fade as the common bond between us grows.

I eat well, drink very little, exercise daily, and laugh as much as I can.

And Jack is still with me. I can't see him, but I feel him. I became "me" with Jack. Nothing can ever take him away. What we shared will always be mine. Finding the strength to build happiness in a new life is an honor to Jack and an honor to our marriage.

Acknowledgements

Just a few weeks after Jack was diagnosed, I sat in our hospital room at Shands watching him as he slept, wondering how I would ever make it through the horror I knew was to come. I was distraught, yet conscious enough to be humiliated by what popped into my mind. "Well, at least I'll be a thin widow." I instantly realized that I needed to talk to others who had gone through this kind of experience. I knew I needed a book to read to confirm that I wasn't a horrible person because of the thoughts that forced themselves upon me. I loved Jack as much as any wife has ever loved her husband, yet *that* is what came to my mind? How can this be? What kind of betrayal is it to know that I'm thinking about my own survival when my husband is facing the end of his life, and all the suffering and pain that accompanies such a horrific disease as his?

There was never any time to join a support group. No other wives of cancer patients were available to whom I could talk. I looked for books but could only find self-help or spiritual themes about the struggles I was facing. I wanted the gut-wrenching reality presented within the verisimilitude of life. And so I recorded my feelings, interactions, and conversations and saved every single medical document from Jack's care because I knew that sooner or later, I would write this book just in case someone else out there was like me and would want to turn to a book to help them survive.

Though I never found a book that could help me deal with our journey, there were people who helped us who I would like to acknowledge.

I owe a debt of gratitude to all of the medical professionals and staff members at Shands and UMMC. I now know from first-hand experience that the people who dedicate their lives to serving others significantly impact the quality of our lives. I would like to extend a special thanks to the 8 East nurses and staff members at Shands who were life-giving and life-saving. They propped me up and taught me what I needed to learn in order to support Jack. They were filled with compassion and expertise. I truly believe they saved me from falling into a deep despair. Dr. Hyland, the team from *Haven Hospice,* and Jack's home PT provider (Matt) also deserve special thanks.

My family and friends who were part of this journey gave me the strength and support I needed to face each day. Without everyone giving all they gave, Jack and I would have had many fewer moments to share. You know who you are and you know I love you.

I thank all the people who provided feedback during the writing of this book – Diane Lee, Xenia Hadjioannou, Bess Altwerger, Morna McNulty, Sue Coburn, Sarah Wolfgang, John and Eileen Rankie, Jeanne So, Carol Waller, Jeff Shelton, Charlie and Jane Rankie, Marcy Friedman, Maureen Maury and Nick Ambulos.

Finally, I would like to thank Denny Taylor and Garn Press. Denny has supported my efforts and respected my need to tell this story. Garn is an independent press giving voice to authors who might otherwise never be heard. Her unselfish dedication to writers and literacy is astounding.

End Notes: Early Detection Can Save Your Life

Cancer is the second most leading cause of death in the US. In 2014 over 224,000 cases of lung cancer were diagnosed and 159,260 people died from the disease. Lung cancer has surpassed breast cancer as the leading cause of cancer-related deaths for women.

Lung cancer screening has progressed in the few years since Jack was diagnosed with Stage Four lung cancer. Medical research has made continuous progress in detecting and treating lung cancer. The guidelines set by the American Cancer Society encourage screening for anyone between the ages of 55 and 79 who is a smoker (or who has quit in the last fifteen years) and has what is called a 30-pack year history. Results from the National Lung Screening Trials indicate "that there were 20% fewer lung cancer deaths in people who received a low-dose CT scan than with a chest x-ray" (www.cancer.org).

I urge everyone to read the information available to them from the American Cancer Society (www.cancer.org), Cancer.Net (http://www.cancer.net/research-and-advocacy/asco-care-and-treatment-recommendations-patients/lung-cancer-screening) and the Centers for Medicare and Medicaid Services (https://www.cms.gov), and to share the information with as many people as possible. Don't stop there. Investigate the National Cancer Institute (NCI) website (www.cancer.gov), one of the most valuable resources for patients and families. Learn about prevention and action that lead to early detection.

The NCI is funded by the National Institutes of Health (NIH), which received an appropriation of $30.14 billion during the 2014 fiscal year. Of the 27 NIH Centers and Institutes, the National Cancer Institute received the largest share of that at budget, $4.95 billion. The advantages of being treated at an NCI Center cannot be overstated – they are the hub of cancer research where the most current breakthroughs in care can be provided, with a better chance for survival and more treatment options, including the possibility of being part of new clinical trials. Screening is crucial – don't wait for symptoms. Do everything possible to avoid the initial diagnosis being one of an advanced stage of the disease.